I0117170

The Quiet Cure:

How Nature Restores What Life Takes Away

DALIA LATIFE

Title: The Quiet Cure:

How Nature Restores What Life Takes Away

Author: Dalia Latife

Published by Pine Tree Press

PINE TREE
PRESS

www.pinetreepress.com

Printed in USA

DEDICATION

In loving memory of my mother,

who didn't speak in poetry,
but moved through life like a force of nature
grounded, fierce, and unshakably true.
She taught me to stand tall like the pines,
to weather storms without apology,
and to find quiet peace in untamed places.
Her strength runs like a river
beneath every word of this book.

ACKNOWLEDGMENTS

This book was written in the quiet moments—between breaths, between deadlines, between the noise of life. And yet, it would not exist without the presence, encouragement, and wisdom of many.

To those who reminded me that stillness is not a luxury, but a lifeline—thank you.

To my family: your love, stories, and strength shaped the lens through which I see the world.

To my daughters: Your strength, wit, and wonder are constant reminders of what truly matters. You inspire me to keep growing, keep listening, and keep showing up.

To my friends who were there for me during the hard times, who reminded me I was not alone, and who held space when I had no words—you offered quiet companionship when I needed it most.

To the forests, oceans, birdsong, and morning light—thank you for reminding me what it means to come home to myself.

And to every reader who picks up this book in search of calm: I hope these words meet you gently, like sunlight through the trees.

CONTENTS

Introduction: The Importance of Nature in Modern Life

We are living in the most connected time in human history—digitally.

We can reach across continents with a click, attend meetings from kitchen tables, and access more information in a day than our ancestors did in a lifetime. And yet, in all this connection, many of us are feeling strangely untethered.

Because while we have linked ourselves to networks, screens, and schedules, we have quietly disconnected from something more essential: the natural world that once grounded us.

The average person now spends more than 90% of their time indoors.

Our daily environments are shaped by artificial light, filtered air, constant background noise, and endless digital input. We navigate buildings instead of landscapes, scroll more than we stroll, and live most of our lives between walls.

Urban living may be fast, efficient, and full of opportunity—but it comes with an invisible cost.

The nervous system is continuously subjected to various stimulus, resulting in sensory overload. The human body, inherently adapted to natural environments and seasonal cycles, seldom receives opportunities to relax, stabilize, or simply exist.

In this fast-paced world, stress has become a default setting.

Anxiety is common. Burnout is praised as ambition. Sleep disorders are normalized. We reach for solutions in the form of medication, wellness apps, productivity tools, anything to keep up. But we often overlook one of the simplest, oldest, and most powerful tools for healing: nature.

A walk among trees. A moment beside water. The scent of rain on warm soil.

These are not just aesthetic pleasures or weekend luxuries. They are biological necessities. Research has confirmed what many cultures have known for generations: time in nature regulates the nervous system, reduces cortisol (the stress hormone), lowers heart rate and blood pressure, improves mood, boosts attention, and restores cognitive function.

It is not just that nature feels good.

It is that nature returns us to balance.

The rustling of leaves. The call of birds. The wind across your skin. These are not background elements—they are messages to your brain: *you are safe now. You can slow down. You can let go.*

This book was born from a simple truth: we were never meant to live fully indoors, divorced from the rhythms of the living world. For most of human history, we moved with the sun, rested with the moon, touched the earth daily, and recognized ourselves as part of something bigger. We belonged to the land.

Today, that relationship has been interrupted—but not lost.

Nature is still within reach.

It might be a mountain trail, a walk through your neighborhood park, a balcony filled with plants, a single flower blooming in the crack of a sidewalk.

It might be five minutes of sky-gazing. Ten minutes with your hands in the soil. A deep breath beside an open window.

In the pages ahead, we will explore how nature soothes and strengthens us—not only through personal experience, but through the lens of science, culture, and ancient wisdom. You will learn about the Japanese practice of forest bathing. The healing power of water. How dirt can elevate mood. Why sunlight, birdsong, and even houseplants can change your mind and body in ways you might not expect.

This is not a book about escaping your life.

It is a book about recalibrating within it. About restoring what we have forgotten but still long for: the feeling of belonging in our own bodies, our own breath, our own environment.

Because nature does not ask you to change who you are.

It simply asks you to come home—to your senses, your rhythm, your stillness. To remember that you were never separated from it.

And in that remembering, you may just find a kind of healing that no screen, pill, or app can offer.

Personal Stories: When Nature Speaks Softly

The Morning Tree

I used to believe that I didn't have time for nature. Between work, kids, and a million emails, even a walk felt indulgent. But during the pandemic, I started drinking my morning cup of tea next to this one tree outside my apartment building. I never noticed it before—just a scraggly tree between concrete slabs. But each day, it changed a little. New buds. Shifting shadows.

I started to realize I was changing too. Those ten minutes a day—just breathing next to something alive—became a ritual. It was not a forest, but it was enough. That tree taught me to notice again. And that noticing became a kind of peace I did not know I needed.

This simple act of pausing by the tree each morning became a form of mindfulness, allowing me to reconnect with the present moment and find tranquility amidst the chaos of daily life.

This daily ritual offered a break from my busy schedule and enhanced my appreciation for nature. It showed that even in urban areas, finding peace and connecting with nature is possible and beneficial.

The River Walk

I used to walk along the river trail only when I was overwhelmed—when the code wouldn't work, when the meetings stacked up, when I couldn't think straight. At first, it was just about movement. But over time, I noticed something deeper happening.

I would start the walk with my shoulders tight and my mind racing. But the sound of the water, the feel of the wind, the sight of ducks gliding by—it all worked like medicine. I would return home differently. Quieter inside. Clearer. Like the river had pulled the clutter out of me. I still walk there almost every day. Not just to de-stress, but to come back to myself. The river trail became more than just a path; it transformed into a sanctuary where I could reconnect with myself. Each step along the winding path allowed me to shed layers of stress and anxiety, replaced by a sense of calm and clarity. The gentle murmur of the flowing water served as a soothing soundtrack, grounding me in the present moment. The rustling leaves and chirping birds provided a natural symphony that eased my racing thoughts.

Gradually, this daily practice transformed into a structured form of walking meditation. As I moved in rhythm with the natural world, I found that my mind settled, and my perspective shifted. Challenges that once seemed insurmountable began to feel manageable, and creative solutions emerged effortlessly. The river, in its constant flow, taught me the value of letting go and moving forward.

Now, even on days when I'm not overwhelmed, I find myself drawn to the trail. It's become a space for reflection, inspiration, and gratitude. Walking along the river isn't just a means to de-stress; it's a way to reconnect with my inner self and the world around me. In the embrace of nature, I've discovered a profound sense of peace and resilience that continues to nourish me daily.

Garden in the Window

When I lost my husband, the silence in our apartment became deafening, and the once comforting walls felt like they were pressing in on me. Each day blurred into the next, and the thought of venturing beyond my doorstep seemed insurmountable. In an attempt to find a semblance of purpose, I brought home a small pot of basil. Its vibrant green leaves and subtle fragrance introduced a spark of life into my stagnant world.

Encouraged by this tiny success, I added a pot of lavender, its soothing scent bringing a sense of calm to my restless nights. Soon, a collection of succulents joined the ensemble, their varied shapes and resilience mirroring my own journey through grief. My windowsill transformed into a miniature garden, a testament to growth and renewal.

Taking care of these plants became a regular activity. The tasks included watering, pruning, and observing new growth. Speaking to them, I shared my thoughts and feelings, finding a nonjudgmental audience in their silent presence. Their steady growth served as a gentle reminder that life continues, even in the aftermath of loss.

This humble garden in my window became more than just a collection of plants; it was a symbol of hope and resilience. Through nurturing them, I began to nurture myself, rediscovering joy in small moments and reclaiming a sense of purpose. They taught me that healing doesn't always come in grand gestures but often in the quiet persistence of life finding a way forward.

The Empty Bench

There was a park on my commute that I passed every day but never entered. It always seemed like something other people had time for—parents with strollers, retired folks reading, teenagers on skateboards. I was too busy, too tired, too behind on everything. But one afternoon, after a long stretch of burnout and back-to-back meetings, I walked in without planning to. I sat down on an empty bench under a tree. I didn't check my phone. I didn't even think. I just sat.

The breeze moved through the leaves. A squirrel darted by. The shadows shifted slowly across the path. Nothing big happened—but something in me let go. Not all at once, but enough to notice that I had been holding too much.

That bench became my reset button. Ten minutes, three times a week. No agenda. Just stillness. It reminded me that I didn't always need a solution—sometimes I just needed space to breathe.

Chapter 1: The Science of Stress Relief

What Stress Does to Us

Stress is an inevitable aspect of daily life. Whether it involves meeting deadlines, navigating traffic, or balancing family and work responsibilities, many individuals find themselves exhausted. However, stress does not merely cause feelings of being overwhelmed; it impacts the entire body.

Stress, at its core, is a survival response. Our ancestors needed it to escape danger— triggering a cascade of hormones that prepared the body to fight, flee, or freeze. But today's stressors aren't life-or-death. They're recurring, subtle, and often inescapable. The inbox is never empty. The noise never stops. And unlike the clear resolution of running from a predator, our modern worries tend to linger without end.

When you are stressed, your body goes into high alert—your heart races, your muscles tense, your breathing gets shallow. It is your body's way of getting ready to deal with something hard or dangerous. That is great if you are running from a bear. Not so great when it is just a full inbox or a disagreement with your boss.

What's worse, our bodies can't always tell the difference. To your nervous system, a packed calendar or unpaid bill might as well be a wild animal. The same ancient biological responses engage, pumping cortisol and adrenaline into your bloodstream, even though the threat is psychological—not physical.

The problem is, we are not giving ourselves enough time to come back down. We stay "on" all day, and sometimes all night too. Over time, that constant pressure can lead to burnout, anxiety, trouble sleeping, and even physical health issues.

We scroll through our phones in bed, reply to emails during dinner, and mentally rehearse tomorrow's to-do list before we've even finished today's. The result? A baseline of constant activation. Our bodies rarely return to equilibrium. And over time, this becomes the new normal—until something inside us begins to fray.

So how do we hit pause and reset?

We start by remembering that we weren't meant to live like this. And nature—calm, wordless, forgiving—offers us a way back.

How Nature Calms Us Down

Nature has a quiet way of calling us home.

Not with noise or urgency, but with whispers—the rustle of leaves dancing in the wind, the steady rhythm of waves folding into shore, the soft scent of pine or rain on warm soil. These are the sounds and smells of stillness reminders that not everything in life moves fast.

There is an intelligence in the natural world—one that moves in cycles instead of schedules. When we attune to that rhythm, we find our own breathing slowing, our senses opening. Researchers call this the "biophilia effect"—our innate, biological connection to the natural world. It's why we feel calmer looking at greenery, why even hospital patients heal faster when they can see trees through a window.

When we step outside, something inside us loosens. The noise in our heads softens. The weight we did not realize we were carrying begins to lift. We stop bracing ourselves, even if just for a moment.

Even brief exposure to green spaces has been shown to reduce cortisol levels, lower blood pressure, and improve mood. It doesn't take a full day in the forest; just a few minutes of intentional presence can begin to shift your physiology.

Nature does not ask anything about us. It does not rush us. It does not care about unread emails or endless to-do lists. Instead, it invites us to pause. To look up. To breathe a little deeper. In those moments, we return—not just to the world around us, but to ourselves.

This return is not abstract. It is sensory. You feel it in the coolness of shade on your skin, the grounded texture of bark under your palm, the way your footsteps land more softly on soil than on concrete. These small shifts signal safety to the nervous system, letting it know it's okay to downregulate.

The more we listen, the more we remember what it feels like to simply be. To watch sunlight filter through branches, to follow the flight of a bird across an open sky, to feel the warmth of a rock beneath our hands. These details, often unnoticed, are nature's way of saying: you are safe, you can let go now.

And that is where the healing begins.

When you are outside, your mind is not spinning in circles. You are not doom-scrolling or overanalyzing. You are watching a bird hop across a path or feeling the sun on your skin. That simplicity helps reset the nervous system and clear mental clutter.

It's not about escape. It's about reconnection. Nature anchors us in the now—away from abstract worries and back into the immediacy of the body.

Why This Matters

We were not designed to live this way—indoors for most of our days, under artificial light, tethered to screens, and bombarded by notifications. Our nervous systems were not built for the pace of modern life, for the constant hum of urgency. Somewhere along the way, we began to treat rest as luxury and stillness as laziness. But nature reminds us that slowing down is not only natural—it is necessary.

We thrive in the sunlight. We steady ourselves quietly. We come alive in open spaces. Our minds crave the gentle rhythms of the natural world, not because it is a nice escape, but because it is where we are wired to feel whole. The fresh air, the rustling trees, the distant sound of birds, these are not background elements. They are medicine for a tired soul.

And here is the beautiful part: it does not have to be dramatic. You do not need a week in the wilderness or a cabin in the woods to feel the effects. Even small, intentional moments—a walk around the block, sitting beneath a tree, tending to a potted plant on your windowsill—can offer real relief. Just a few minutes of presence, surrounded by something alive and growing, can shift your day.

Microdoses of nature have macro impact. In Japan, researchers developed the practice of "shinrin-yoku," or forest bathing, after discovering how time in wooded areas significantly lowered stress hormone levels and improved immune function. Their findings continue to influence wellness models around the world.

The more we understand how stress affects our bodies and minds, the more we realize how simple the antidote can be. Nature gives freely. We only have to remember to receive it.

Because sometimes, the most effective form of therapy is not found in a bottle or an app. Sometimes, it is simply found outside your door.

Chapter 2: Forest Bathing & Biophilia

Forest Bathing Across Cultures: Global Practices, Shared Roots

Long before "forest bathing" became a trending wellness practice, people across the world had already been turning to trees, trails, and stillness for healing. The method may differ by name or ritual, but the intention is shared: to restore the human spirit through deep connection with the natural world.

While Japan's *Shinrin-yoku* is the most widely known, it is only one branch of a much older, much broader tree.

Shinrin-yoku: Breathing in the Forest

In the early 1980s, Japan was facing a quiet crisis. The economy was booming, but people were burning out. Work culture was intense, stress-related illnesses were rising, and citizens were growing increasingly disconnected from the natural beauty that surrounded them. In response, the Japanese Ministry of Forestry introduced a simple yet profound concept: Shinrin-yoku, or *forest bathing.*

But forest bathing is not about exercise. You are not jogging or hiking. There is no goal, no step count, no performance. Instead, it is about immersion—being present in the forest with all your senses. You walk slowly, breathe deeply, listen carefully. You take in the scent of the trees, the feel of the breeze on your skin, the dappled light filtering through branches. It is not a workout. It is a waking meditation in nature.

Japanese researchers began studying its effects and the results were compelling. People who practiced Shinrin-yoku had lower cortisol levels, reduced heart rates, and improved moods. Their immune systems were stronger, showing increased activity in natural killer (NK) cells—critical for fighting infections and even cancer. The forests were not just pretty, they were medicinal.

Today, Japan has dozens of officially designated forest therapy trails, and the practice has spread worldwide. But you do not need to fly to a cedar grove in Kyoto to experience it. A quiet park, a stand of trees, even a small garden can offer a space for stillness and restoration.

At its heart, Shinrin-yoku is about slowing down enough to let nature in—not just as a backdrop, but as a participant in your healing.

South Korea – Healing Forests and Government Support

Inspired by Japan's *Shinrin-yoku* and motivated by rising mental health concerns, South Korea has taken forest therapy a step further by integrating it into national policy. The government has established over thirty designated "healing forests" (치유의 숲, *Chiyu-ui Sup*) across the country, many of them near major urban centers like Seoul and Busan, making nature-based healing more accessible than ever before.

These forests are not simply preserved—they are purposefully designed for restoration. Each healing forest includes certified trails tailored to different physical abilities, dedicated zones for rest and meditation, and often on-site wellness centers staffed by trained professionals. These centers offer services such as aromatherapy, nature-based art therapy, forest sound immersion, and guided breathing sessions among trees.

There is even an official profession known as forest healing instructors, who are trained to lead individuals and groups through practices that slow the body and calm the mind. These guides do more than offer walks—they facilitate intentional connection with the land, often blending ancient wisdom with modern therapeutic methods.

Nature as Communal Medicine

Unlike some Western practices that emphasize solitary reflection, Korean forest healing is often experienced together. Communal walks, shared silence, and group meditation form the heart of many programs. There is a quiet understanding that healing is not just internal, but relational—we reconnect with ourselves *and* with each other through the land.

Participants are guided through deeply sensory experiences:

- "Forest breathing," where you inhale deeply beneath tall pines, synchronizing breath with movement.
- Silent walking meditations, often in a single line, feeling the ground through every step.
- Hands-on engagement with natural textures, such as pinecones, bark, or moss
- Reflection circles after walks, where stories and emotions are shared gently, often over tea brewed with forest herbs.

This structure reflects a cultural value rooted in harmony—with nature, with family, with community. It is not simply about the individual's recovery; it is about restoring the whole.

A Response to a Changing World

Forest therapy in South Korea also speaks to a deeper national need. As urbanization, academic pressure, and work stress continue to weigh heavily on the population, particularly among youth and older adults, the healing forests serve as a **counterbalance to modern life**.

Special programs are tailored for groups who have experienced trauma, such as **first responders, veterans, and survivors of domestic violence**. Others support **students overwhelmed by academic pressure**, or elders who deal with loneliness and grief. For each group, the forest becomes more than a setting—it becomes **a source of refuge and renewal.**

Healing Through the Seasons

Korean healing forests are accessible throughout the year, with seasonal changes enhancing the experience. In spring, the trails are adorned with blooming azaleas and cherry blossoms. During summer, visitors can enjoy cool, shaded areas beneath the tall fir trees. Autumn's golden forests invite reflection and letting go. And in winter, quiet snowcovered paths encourage deep rest and stillness.

Each season, like each walk, offers its own kind of medicine.

The Forest as a Cultural Healer

In South Korea, the rise of healing forests is not just a wellness trend—it is a cultural evolution. It reflects an increasing understanding: **that healing can occur not only through clinical treatment or discussions, but also through the natural environment, such as the sound of leaves, the scent of pine, and the experience of silence** under the sky.

The forest is not a retreat from life.

It is a return to something ancient, sacred, and quietly powerful.

Finland & the Nordic Countries – Nature as a Way of Life In Finland, nature is not a destination. It is a companion.

The forest is not something to schedule or escape to—it is simply part of life, woven into daily routines, language, memory, and identity. there is a word in Finnish that captures this beautifully: **Metsän Lumo**— *"the enchantment of the forest."* It refers to the spell that nature casts when you allow yourself to enter it fully, not as a visitor, but as something that belongs.

Here, **forest bathing is not a named practice—it is a way of being**.

You will find people of all ages walking alone in the woods, not for exercise or a goal, but for quiet. It is not unusual to see someone lying back in a bed of moss, eyes closed, listening to the wind. **There is no need for instruction, no pressure to be mindful. The forest teaches presence simply by being itself.**

Everyday Rituals, Quietly Sacred

Nature is integrated into Finnish life with simplicity and reverence.

- Families spend weekends at forest cabins, known as mökki, often without electricity or running water.
- Children are taught from an early age to play outside in all weather, learning not just resilience, but the relationship with the land.
- Foraging is a cherished tradition—picking wild blueberries, gathering wild herbs, nettles, or rose hips is not seen as rare—it is a natural part of living in tune with the land's quiet offerings.
- Many take breaks during workday to walk through green spaces or simply sit beneath trees, letting the stillness recalibrate their nervous systems.

Nature is not considered a luxury here. It is not something to earn.

It is **a basic human right**, even written into law. In Finland and much of the Nordic region, the principle of **"Everyman's Right" (*jokamiehenoikeus*)** grants all people the freedom to roam forests, lakes, and meadows—regardless of who owns the land.

It is a cultural belief that **nature belongs to everyone**, and that everyone belongs to nature.

The Forest as a Place of Mental Recovery

Finland's deep integration with nature is not just romantic—it is practical.

With long, dark winters and some of the highest reported rates of seasonal depression in Europe, the country has embraced green spaces as a form of public health.

Research from Finnish universities shows that spending as little as **15 minutes in a natural environment**—a park, trail, or tree-lined street—can lower cortisol levels, reduce feelings of anxiety, and restore focus. These effects are especially notable in urban dwellers, who are often surrounded by noise, concrete, and sensory overload.

In Helsinki, city planning prioritizes **access to nearby forests and lakes**, ensuring that even residents in dense neighborhoods are no more than a short walk from trees and water.

Here, the forest is not an antidote to burnout. It is **the buffer that prevents it.**

More Than Wellness—A Way of Remembering

For the people of Finland and the wider Nordic world, nature is not something to escape into. It is something to come home to.

It does not require apps or subscriptions or guided walks. It only asks that you step into it—and listen.

The moss will cushion your thoughts.

The trees will hold your silence.

The wind will speak to what you have forgotten.

And in that stillness, you will remember something true:

You are part of the forest.

You are not lost.

You are returning.

Biophilia: Our Inborn Love of Nature

Why does forest bathing feel so natural—so deeply comforting—even to those who have never heard of it before?

That is where the idea of biophilia comes in.

Coined by biologist E.O. Wilson, biophilia suggests that humans have an innate emotional connection to nature—a deep-rooted affinity that comes from millennia of living alongside trees, rivers, animals, and open skies. We evolved outdoors. For 99% of human history, survival depended on reading the land, listening to the wind, watching the sky. Nature was not something we visited on weekends; it was home.

Even today, our bodies recognize nature as familiar ground. Studies from Japan, Finland, Sweden, and the U.S. show related results: time in green spaces reduces anxiety, boosts mood, sharpens focus, and encourages creativity. Finnish researchers found that just 15 minutes in a park can significantly improve mood and attention. In Sweden, hospital patients with views of trees recovered faster than those facing walls. In the UK, doctors are prescribing time in nature alongside traditional treatment for depression and high blood pressure.

There is something quietly profound about that: a walk in the woods can be as therapeutic as a pill.

The Forest Is Not a Luxury, it is a Lifeline.

In fast-paced, noisy cities, green space often feels like a luxury—something extra. But research and ancient wisdom alike show us that it is a necessity. We do not just like nature. We need it. It calms the nervous system, deepens breath, restores perspective. It reminds us that there is more to life than our inbox, more to us than what we produce.

Forest bathing and biophilia both teach the same lesson in diverse ways: we are not separate from nature—we are part of it. When we spend time outside, we are not escaping the real world. We are entering it.

So, the next time you feel tense, scattered, or overwhelmed, consider stepping outside— not to escape, but to remember.

Look up into the trees. Listen to the wind. Breathe like the forest is breathing with you. Let your thoughts slow to the rhythm of rustling leaves. Let your heartbeat soften to the pulse of the earth beneath your feet.

Notice the way sunlight flickers through branches, how shadows stretch and shrink across the path.

Let the cool air touch your skin like a quiet reassurance: *you are here, you are alive, and you are part of this.* there is no pressure to fix anything. No one to impress. No urgency beyond this moment.

In the forest, there is no judgment. Only invitation.

An invitation to stop striving, to stop bracing, to stop apologizing for being tired.

Here, you are enough—as you are.

Closing Reflection: Returning to the Forest

The forest does not demand that you understand it.

It does not ask for achievement, productivity, or certainty.

It only asks that you arrive—with open senses and an unclenched heart.

Whether you walk in silence beneath tall pines or sit near the rustling edge of a city tree, something quiet begins to happen. You begin to *remember.* Not with your mind, but with your body—with your breath, your skin, your slowing pulse.

You remember that peace does not always come in answers.

Sometimes it comes in presence.

Sometimes, in the hush between wind gusts.

Sometimes, in the way sunlight moves through leaves like water.

Across cultures, landscapes, and histories, people have turned to the forest—not as escape, but as return. A return to rhythm. A return to relationship. A return to what is real.

This is not a practice reserved for others. You don't need special training or perfect weather or a map to find your way. The path to stillness is not paved with instructions. It is marked by awareness.

Step outside. Let the forest greet you as you are.

Not as someone trying to heal, but as someone who is already part of the healing. Already part of the earth's slow exhale.

Because when you spend time among trees—really *spend* time—you are not just observing nature.

You are being reabsorbed by it.

And in that quiet reunion, something sacred happens:

You remember that you belong.

Chapter 3: The Role of Light, Air, and Sound

Sometimes, it is not just what we see in nature that soothes us—it is what we feel, hear, and breathe. Long before we had words for anxiety or terms like "burnout," our bodies were responding to subtle shifts in the environment—light warming the skin, the crispness of morning air, the sound of wind moving through trees. These are not just sensory details; they are deeply restorative experiences that speak directly to the nervous system.

Sunlight and Fresh Air: Nature's Gentle Wake-Up Call

There is something undeniably calming about standing in the sun with your eyes closed, your face tilted upward, letting the light wash over you. That is not just a nice moment, it is chemistry. Natural sunlight helps regulate our circadian rhythms, the internal clock that governs sleep, mood, and energy. When we get sunlight, especially in the morning—it signals to the brain: wake up, feel alert, get moving.

Sunlight also triggers the release of serotonin, often called the "feel-good" hormone. Higher serotonin levels are linked to improved mood and a sense of calm focus. That is why just 10–15 minutes of sun exposure can make such a noticeable difference, especially after time indoors.

And then there is fresh air, cool, clean, unprocessed. It carries moisture, earthy scents, and invisible compounds released by plants and trees. Inhaling this kind of air is different than the stale, recycled air of an office or crowded building. It is richer in oxygen and often infused with phytoncides, natural substances emitted by trees known to lower stress hormones and support immune health.

Together, sunlight and fresh air are like nature's reset button—offered to us every day if we only step outside to receive it.

Practical Tips for Urban Settings:

- Spend the first 10 minutes of your day outside or by a sunlit window.
- Take short walks around the block during lunch.
- Keep houseplants near windows to bridge indoor and outdoor air quality.
- Open windows daily to circulate fresh air, even briefly.
- Work near natural light sources when possible.
- Natural Soundscapes: The Music of Calm

Close your eyes and imagine this: The slow ripple of water brushing against the shore. Birds calling softly in the distance. Leaves whispering overhead as the wind weaves gently through the trees. You breathe in, slowly. And for a moment—there is only calm.

Now contrast that with the sharp blare of a car horn. The persistent ding of a phone notification. The low hum of traffic and the distant rise of a siren echoing between buildings. One environment invites your nervous system to soften. The other asks it to stay alert.

Sound plays a powerful, often invisible role in how we feel. Even when we are not consciously aware of it, our bodies are always listening. They are attuned to the world around us, scanning for cues: Are we safe? Are we at ease? Or should we be ready to react?

Natural soundscapes—like the rustling of leaves, the flow of a stream, rainfall on a rooftop, or ocean waves folding into the shore—have been shown to reduce stress, lower heart rate, and promote focus. A study found that individuals who listened to nature sounds through headphones performed better on memory tasks and reported feeling calmer and more grounded than those exposed to urban noise or silence.

Why is that? Because natural sounds follow a rhythm we instinctively understand. They rise and fall gently. They are soft but not silent, full but not overwhelming. They mirror the patterns of our breath, our heartbeat, our thoughts when they are not being pulled in a dozen directions.

Urban environments, on the other hand, often bombard us with sudden, sharp, high pitched sounds. Sirens. Alarms. Horns. Even the background hum of electricity or traffic can subtly activate our stress response. These are the kinds of noises that the nervous system registers as a potential threat even if we have learned to ignore them on the surface. But underneath? The body is still responding. Still tense. Still staying alert.

That is why even when you cannot access a forest or beach in person, simply listening to recordings of nature can begin to shift your physiology. The sound of rain, a crackling fire, or waves rolling in—these are more than ambiance. These are invitations that encourage the body to remember and revert to a slower, familiar rhythm. It is a pace the body is well acquainted with and eagerly seeks to experience once again.

Practical Tips for Tuning In:

- Use nature sound playlists or apps during work, rest, or meditation.
- Keep a small indoor water fountain for ambient sound.
- Visit green spaces with water features, even in city parks.
- Choose quiet, green walking routes over busy streets when possible.
- Schedule five-minute "sound breaks" throughout

your day with bird song or soft rain.

Why These Elements Matter

Sunlight. Fresh air. The soft hush of leaves moving in the wind. These elements may seem small—ordinary, even—but they carry a quiet power that our bodies instinctively recognize. They do not demand our attention. They do not flash, ping, or scroll. Instead, they arrive gently, asking nothing of us but our presence.

In a world that constantly competes for our focus, that kind of subtlety can be easy to overlook. We are conditioned to value what is loud, fast, and productive. But nature speaks in a different language—one that soothes instead of stimulates. One that does not overwhelm but restores.

The warmth of the sun on your skin is not just pleasant. It signals your body to release serotonin, lifts your mood, and regulates your sleep cycle. A deep breath of fresh air does not just feel clean—it is. It is rich in oxygen and scent, a subtle reset for your nervous system. The gentle sound of birdsong or rustling trees reminds your brain that you are safe, that the world is not always urgent, that peace is possible even in motion.

These natural elements form the invisible atmosphere that supports well-being—not through effort, but through simplicity.

They bring us back to what is real: The rise and fall of the sun. The inhale and exhale of wind. The rhythm of rain, the rustle of leaves, the dance of light through trees.

No Wi-Fi required. No app to install. No steps to master. Just presence. Just being.

In this overstimulated world, where screens glow late into the night and every silence seems to beg for filling, these natural elements remind us of what it means to be human. Not just functioning. Not just producing. But living—embodied, breathing, aware.

They bring us back to the moment. Back to the body. Back to the earth. And most importantly, they remind us that we are not separate from the world around us. We are not machines wired to run endlessly. We are nature too. And when we allow ourselves to return to its rhythm—even briefly—we remember what it feels like to be whole.

Closing Reflection

The next time you feel foggy, restless, or overwhelmed, pause before reaching for another cup of coffee or scrolling through your phone. Not because those things are wrong—but because they may not give you what you truly need.

Instead, open a window. Step outside, even if just for a moment. Feel the air shift against your skin. Find a patch of sunlight and breathe it in. Let the breeze move across your face. Listen—not for anything specific, but for whatever is there: the rustle of leaves, distant birdsong, the sound of your own breath settling.

You don't need a forest to feel relief.

You don't need an hour to feel calm.

You just need a moment of attention—a break in the noise—to let your body remember what safety and presence feel like.

Nature doesn't speak in commands. It won't fix your to-do list or erase your stress. But it offers something far more sustainable: a different pace. A steady rhythm. A place to come back to when the world feels too much.

Let the natural world remind you—quietly, and without needing to say anything—that you are part of something softer, slower, and more enduring than stress.

You are not disconnected.

You are not behind.

You are simply tired. And nature knows how to hold that.

Return to the wind. To sunlight. To soil.

Let them do what they've always done:

Support you. Settle you. Welcome you home.

Chapter 4: Blue Spaces: The Healing Power of Water

There is a reason we are drawn to water.

We walk along the ocean's edge just to hear the waves. We pause at rivers, let fountains hold our gaze, sit silently beside lakes without needing to speak. Water does not rush us. It invites us to breathe slower, to listen, to feel something settle within us.

It is hard to explain, but we know it when we feel it—that deep exhale that comes when we are near water. That quiet comfort that says *you are okay. Just be here.*

There is a name for this: **Blue Mind**, coined by marine biologist Dr. Wallace J. Nichols. It describes the calm, meditative state that water environments evoke—a contrast to the "red mind" of anxiety and stimulation that modern life often demands. When we are near water, our brains shift into a more relaxed mode, easing stress and inviting clarity.

Why Water Feels Like Home

Water has always been part of us.

Before we ever opened our eyes, before we spoke or stood or knew the weight of the world, we floated—cradled in warmth, in rhythm, in fluid motion. We were surrounded by it, sustained by it. We came into being through it.

Maybe that is why, even now, being near water feels like a kind of memory.

It does not have to be the vastness of the ocean. A still pond, a winding creek, the gentle trickle of a stream in the woods—any of it can stir something in us. Something ancestral. Something instinctual. A quiet recognition that this is where life begins, and this is where we return when we are trying to feel whole again.

There is a subtle shift that happens near water. Our shoulders drop. Our breath deepens. The noise in our heads starts to fade. We do not have to work at it—it just happens, as if our bodies know what to do in the presence of this ancient element.

Even the sound of water—gentle waves, soft rainfall, the echo of a distant splash—creates a kind of peace we do not realize we have been missing until it is there. These sounds speak directly to the nervous system, guiding us back to calm, back to presence, back to ourselves.

This isn't just poetic—it's physiological. Research shows that natural water sounds can help reduce cortisol levels, lower blood pressure, and even synchronize brain waves into more restful patterns. Our bodies remember what stillness feels like when they are near water. We don't have to try. We simply respond.

Water Teaches Us How to Let Go

Water has a way of holding space without holding on.

Rivers do not pause to question what they carry. They move—fluidly, easily, accepting and releasing in the same breath.

The ocean never resists the tide. It rises and recedes, collecting and surrendering in one graceful motion.

Rain falls without apology. Lakes reflect without judgment. Streams make music out of movement.

And in this, water offers us something profound: *permission to release.*

When life feels heavy—when your mind is cluttered, or your heart feels like it is carrying too much—water, does not try to fix it.

It does not ask questions. It does not demand answers. It simply is—steady, accepting, alive.

Sit beside it long enough, and you might notice your thoughts loosening, the tension in your chest easing.

Not because you solved anything, but because you were finally given space to soften.

Water teaches us that letting go is not weakness.

It is flow.

It is trust.

It is the choice to stop gripping and allow things to move through us—grief, fear, hope, longing—without resistance.

It reminds us that we can begin again. With every ripple. Every drop. Every tide.

And maybe, with every return to water, we remember that we do not need to hold it all alone.

You Do Not Need the Ocean

You do not need to travel far to feel this shift.

You do not need a week-long retreat or a mountaintop lake.

Sometimes, peace comes in smaller forms:

- A neighborhood pond where ducks glide across glassy water.
- A city fountain trickling beneath the noise of passing cars.
- The warm rhythm of a shower after a long day.
- Rain tapping gently on your windowsill while you pause in silence.

Even a bowl of water with floating petals on your desk can

bring you back to stillness. A reminder. A symbol. A quiet touchpoint with something ancient and elemental.

It is not about the scale of the water—it is about the invitation it offers:

To slow down.

To soften.

To sit still and let your thoughts settle, like silt drifting to the bottom of a stream.

You do not need to go to the ocean to feel what water can do.

You only need to notice it. To be with it. To let it be what it always is—patient, powerful, and deeply, deeply healing.

Water is one of the oldest mirrors we have—reflecting both the sky above and the stillness we carry within.

Closing Reflection

When the world feels loud and your heart feels full of things you can't quite name, go to the water.

Let it cradle your weariness without needing to fix it.

Let it take your unspoken questions and carry them downstream. Let it show you how to soften—without breaking.

Watch the ripples stretch, the current flow, the stillness in between. You do not have to have answers here. You only have to be.

Because healing is not always found in effort. Sometimes, it arrives in the quiet— in the presence of water, in the return to yourself.

Simple Nature Ritual: A Water Release

What you will need: A small bowl of water, a leaf or slip of paper, a pen (optional), and a quiet moment.

1. Sit with your bowl of water. Place your hand above it and take a few slow breaths.
2. Reflect on something you would like to release—an emotion, a thought, a weight you have been carrying.
3. Write it down on the paper or speak it silently into the water.
4. Place the paper or leaf in the bowl and watch it float. Let your release become part of the water.
5. If outdoors, gently pour water into the earth. If indoors, hold the bowl a moment longer before discarding with intention.
6. Close with a hand to your heart and a whispered reminder: *"I am allowed to let go."*

Chapter 5: Attention Restoration Theory

There is a kind of tiredness that sleep does not fix.

It is the mental fog that builds from decision after decision, from scrolling through endless information, from navigating noise, traffic, deadlines, and demands. It is the feeling of being mentally "on" all the time—focused, alert, overstimulated—and somehow still unable to concentrate on what really matters.

We often call it burnout, but long before it gets that far, it is something simpler: cognitive fatigue. A brain that is just... tired of paying attention.

And this is where nature offers something incredibly powerful—not just rest, but restoration.

Restoring Focus and Mental Clarity

Most of us think of rest as doing nothing: sitting on the couch, turning off the lights, maybe taking a nap or binging a show. And while physical rest matters, it does not always restore the *mind*. Sometimes, even after a break, we still feel scattered, foggy, or disconnected.

Nature helps in a different way. It does not just give the brain a break—it gives it something better to do.

This is the quiet magic of attention restored—not forced, not rushed, simply invited. Nature does not demand your focus; it gently holds it. A drifting cloud, the sway of a tree, the shimmer of a waterfall of it holds your attention gently, without demand.

It is not about shutting off your thoughts. It is about giving them space to breathe, wander, and return home.

Why?

Because nature offers what they call "soft fascination." In other words, the sights and sounds of nature are interesting enough to hold our attention, but not so intense that they drain it. A fluttering leaf, a rippling stream, clouds drifting across the sky, these moments pull us in just enough to quiet the noise inside, without demanding anything from us.

It is a kind of effortless attention that gives our minds space to wander, sort, and eventually, return.

Urban vs. Natural Environments

Now think about a typical day in the city or even a suburban neighborhood. Traffic lights, sirens, screens, crowded sidewalks, multitasking are all examples of what researchers call directed attention, and it requires effort. You have to filter out distractions, stay alert, make choices, and constantly shift focus.

Over time, this wears the brain down. You might notice it in little ways, forgetting why you walked into a room, rereading the same paragraph over and over, or feeling like your thoughts are running on empty.

Natural environments, on the other hand, do the opposite. They do not overload the senses; they soothe them. You do not have to filter loud noises or flashing ads. You can just *be.* In fact, studies have shown that people who spend time in green spaces—even for a short while—score higher on tests measuring memory, creativity, and sustained attention.

Everyday Restoration

You do not need a weekend retreat or a mountain view to benefit from attention restoration. A walk in the park. Sitting by a window with a view of trees. Watching the sky change colors as the sun sets. Even just a few mindful minutes outside can help clear mental fog and make space for new ideas to flow.

The key is to let go of trying to be productive while you are out there. Let nature take the lead. Let your eyes wander, your thoughts drift. Let your focus unspool and slowly return on its own.

How This Works in Everyday Life

In Schools: Supporting Focus and Learning

Children today face growing academic pressure and decreasing outdoor time. Classrooms are often packed with visual clutter, harsh lighting, noise, and rigid structures, all of which tax their ability to focus and self-regulate. Attention spans shrink under constant stimulation and structured demands, and many children experience burnout long before their school day ends.

Nature offers a counterbalance.

Even short exposure to green spaces has been shown to significantly boost attention and reduce behavioral issues. In Finland and other Nordic countries, schools incorporate outdoor lessons, nature walks, and unstructured play into the school day—not as a break from learning, but as an integral part of it. Research shows that students who learn in natural environments show improved memory, better test performance, and greater emotional resilience.

A school does not need to be in the forest to benefit. Small steps—like placing plants in classrooms, adding outdoor seating areas, or creating sensory gardens—can make a profound difference. Teachers can guide students in silent nature walks, journaling under trees, or even short visualizations using nature soundscapes inside the classroom.

When the school environment shifts to support restoration, not just output—students feel it. They focus better. They relate more calmly. And they begin to understand that learning does not just happen at a desk, it happens in the quiet attention of a leaf, the stillness of a shadow, the rhythm of a breeze.

Nature does not replace education. It **restores the minds** that education depends on.

How nature helps:

- Classrooms with views of trees or natural light see improved test scores and behavior.
- A 15-minute recess in a green space significantly aids students in returning to their activities with increased focus and calmness.
- "Outdoor classrooms" and nature-based curriculums boost memory, problemsolving, and engagement.

Try this:

- Add a nature corner to classrooms with leaves, stones, or plants students can observe.
- Integrate short "green breaks"—2–5 minutes of nature visuals or soundscapes between lessons.
- Encourage barefoot time on grass, sketching outdoors, or even cloud-watching to bring stillness into learning.

In Workplaces:

Restoring Creative Energy and Mental Clarity

Office life often means staring at screens for hours, surrounded by artificial lighting, digital noise, and an unrelenting stream of tasks and notifications. The result? Mental fatigue, diminished creativity, and emotional depletion.

Our brains were not designed to operate in constant output mode. Without intentional moments of rest, the quality of focus and clarity begins to fray. That is where nature—even in small doses—becomes essential.

Research shows that employees who have access to natural views or incorporate nature into their workday experience lower stress levels, increased productivity, and enhanced problem-solving abilities. A brief walk outside, a few minutes near a window, or a meeting held in a courtyard can all provide the kind of soft fascination that allows the mind to reset.

Workplaces can support this by incorporating biophilic design—adding plants, natural textures, open windows, or calming nature sounds. Simple shifts, like relocating break areas to sunny, green-adjacent spots or encouraging walking meetings outdoors, can transform a company culture from burnout-driven to wellness-aligned.

Even in remote work settings, personalizing a workspace with elements of nature—a few houseplants, a bowl of stones, a landscape print, or a natural sound playlist—can help restore balance.

Nature does not ask us to do more. It invites us to pause, breathe, and return to our work with a renewed sense of presence.

Because creativity does not thrive in pressure. It blooms in space. And nature knows exactly how to make space for us.

How nature helps:

- Views of greenery or walking meetings in natural settings improve concentration and reduce error rates.
- Nature imagery and indoor plants have been shown to lower stress and enhance cognitive flexibility.
- Employees who take short breaks outdoors are more productive and less emotionally drained.

Try this:

- Place your desk near a window, or display landscape photos on your screen.
- Take 10-minute "micro-walks" outside after high-

focus tasks.

- Use nature-based break zones—benches in courtyards, rooftop gardens, or even plant-filled rooms—to create mental reset spaces.

At Home: Reclaiming Focus in Everyday Spaces

Whether you work from home, care for others, or simply try to rest at the end of a long day, your home can become a place of background stress. Laundry piles. Notifications. Artificial light late into the night. Constant mental tabs open—even if the room is quiet.

Over time, this ambient tension builds up. It wears down our ability to focus, rest, or feel restored in the very place meant to shelter us. But by inviting nature into our living spaces, we can transform the atmosphere without changing our entire routine.

Even small interactions with nature—a few minutes on a balcony, watering a plant, opening a window to hear birds or rain—can reset our overstimulated systems. These moments work not because they solve our to-do lists, but because they reconnect with a rhythm outside of urgency.

Greenery softens the room. Natural light shifts mood. The scent of soil, the sound of wind, or the sight of sky can offer a calming cue to your nervous system: *you can rest here.*

Nature-based practices at home can be incredibly simple:

- Start the day with a breath at an open window.
- Take a grounding break with a walk around the block or time in a backyard.
- Turn a corner of your space into a "nature nook" with plants, stones, or light.

- Listen to nature's soundscapes while cooking or cleaning.
- Dim artificial lighting in the evening and use candlelight to mimic the setting sun.

You do not need a forest to restore your focus. You just need intention—and a few moments to let nature meet you where you are.

Because in the stillness of leaves, in the coolness of morning air, in the flicker of sunlight through a window, there is something deeply familiar: a reminder that home is not just where we live.

It is where we **return to ourselves.**

How nature helps:

- Short periods of nature exposure—through windows, balconies, gardens—restore attention even more effectively than rest alone.
- Time spent tending a plant, watching the sky, or listening to outdoor sounds can quiet the mind and reduce mental clutter.
- Children in homes with more green space show stronger self-regulation and emotional control.

Try this:

- Begin and end your day with five minutes near a window or outdoors.
- Create a nature nook: a chair by a window, a candle by a plant, or a spot to sip tea and look at the sky.
- Open a window and journal beside it—even the view of trees or clouds can begin to restore your focus.

Closing Reflection

Your mind is not a machine.

It is a living, changing, sensitive part of you that sometimes needs stillness to remember how to think clearly again.

So, the next time you feel scattered, stuck, or unfocused, step outside.

Let the trees do the talking. Let the wind sort through your thoughts.

Let the world remind you that clarity does not always come from pushing harder. Sometimes, it comes from looking at the sky and remembering how to pause.

Chapter 6: Digital Detox Outdoors

There is a special kind of exhaustion that creeps in when we have spent too long behind a screen. It is not always physical, but it is heavy. Our eyes ache. Our thoughts feel scrambled. Our emotions run shallow, or not at all. Even when we are still, our minds do not feel still. This is the quiet toll of digital fatigue—a kind of burnout we rarely name yet deeply feel.

We reach for our phones first thing in the morning and carry them with us until we fall asleep. We check email while walking, scroll while eating, and absorb more information in a single day than generations before us ever did in a week. And yet, the more we consume, the less full we feel.

That is where nature comes in—not as a luxury, but as a remedy.

The Weight of Constant Input

Our digital world is loud—even when it is silent. Each ping, notification, or flashing screen keeps our nervous system on high alert. It is not just the content that drains us, it is the *constant* shift in attention. A news headline, a message, a meme, a memory within seconds. Our brains were not built for this kind of multitasking marathon.

This level of constant engagement leads to mental fatigue, emotional dullness, and decision overload. It becomes harder to focus, harder to connect, harder to feel grounded.

That is when nature steps in with something radically different: nothing to click, nothing to scroll, nothing to "catch up on."

Why Nature Works as a Reset

Spending time outside helps reset the nervous system. It offers a slower rhythm that our minds instinctively remember. Trees do not rush. Clouds do not demand a reply. A quiet trail does not ask anything of you but your presence.

Where screens pull our attention in a hundred directions, nature gently invites it back to the moment. This is the magic of a digital detox outside, not just unplugging but reconnecting with what is real and restorative.

Nature calms the senses:

- Eyes soften with distant views and natural light.
- Ears relax with the hush of wind or birdsong.
- Hands remember the feel of rough bark or cool stone.
- The mind stops scanning for updates and begins to rest.

Even a short walk without a phone can shift your energy. A day away from screens, spent under trees or near water, can feel like a reset you did not know you needed.

Small Detoxes, Big Impact

You do not need to go off the grid to experience the benefits. Try simple rituals:

- A walk without headphones
- Eating one meal a day outdoors
- Leaving your phone inside while sitting on the porch
- Replacing one scroll session with sky-watching or cloud gazing

What you will often find is this: the less noise you make, the more you can hear your own thoughts.

A Step-by-Step Guide

In a world that moves at the speed of a swipe, being constantly connected can come at a cost. Screens keep us informed and engaged—but they also keep our nervous systems alert and overloaded. A digital detox outdoors offers a chance to slow down, reconnect, and restore your attention span by turning away from devices and toward the natural world.

Here is a gentle, step-by-step guide to creating your own digital detox experience:

Step 1: Set Your Intention

Before turning off your phone, pause. Ask yourself: *What am I hoping to gain from this break?* Clarity? Calm? Presence? Let this intention guide you through the process.

Step 2: Choose a Timeframe

Start small. Even 30 minutes away from screens can be healing. As you grow more comfortable, extend the window to a full morning, afternoon, or weekend.

Step 3: Pick Your Place

Find a spot in nature—a park, trail, beach, garden, or even your backyard. Choose somewhere that allows you to observe, breathe, and move without digital interruption.

Step 4: Power Down

Silence your devices. Better yet, turn them off or leave them behind. If safety is a concern, keep your phone on airplane mode in your bag.

Step 5: Tune Into Your Senses

Notice what you hear, see, feel, and smell. Let your senses guide you. Walk slowly. Sit under a tree. Breathe in the scent of soil or pine. Feel the ground beneath your feet.

Step 6: Let Go of Expectations

You do not have to come back with answers. There is no productivity metric here. Your only job is to be present.

Step 7: Reflect Afterward

Take a few moments after your detox to journal, sketch, or simply sit in stillness. Ask: *What did I notice without my screen? What did I feel? What do I want to remember?*

Optional Enhancements:

- Bring a small nature journal.
- Create a simple ritual (lighting a candle, sipping tea)
- Invite a friend to join you in silence.
- Pair your detox with grounding exercises like barefoot walking or nature-based meditation.

Closing Reflection

When life feels too fast, too full, too loud—go outside.

Leave the device behind. Step into a space where nothing is curated, nothing is filtered, and everything is real.

Let the trees remind you what stillness feels like.

Let the sky remind you how to look up. Let the wind carry away the static.

Because sometimes, healing is not about doing less, it is about being present with more of what matters.

Chapter 7:
Designing a Nature Routine

You do not need a cabin in the woods to feel connected to nature.

You do not need hiking boots or hours of free time.

You just need intentions and a little room to breathe.

Even the smallest acts—like noticing the way light touches your windowsill or pausing to listen to the wind—can become gateways back to presence. Nature doesn't ask for grandeur. It asks for attention. And by offering it, we often find that we receive far more than we expected.

In a world that fills our calendars, drains our batteries, and pulls our focus in a dozen directions, building a nature routine is not about escape. It is about return. A return to your senses. A return to rhythm. A return to what grounds you.

It is not about doing more. It is about being more aware. More rooted. More aligned with what restores you instead of what depletes you.

This chapter is about creating space for nature in your everyday life—whether you live in a quiet suburb, a city high-rise, or somewhere in between.

No matter where you are, nature can meet you there.

Why Routine Matters

Just like drinking water or brushing your teeth, being in nature is something your mind and body need regularly—not occasionally. When nature becomes part of your routine, it shifts from something "extra" to something essential. The benefits—calm, clarity, energy, presence—start to compound. And slowly, you begin to feel more rooted, more balanced, more you.

This is how restoration becomes part of your baseline instead of something you seek only when you're burned out. When you integrate nature into your routine, it becomes a quiet partner in your day—not a luxury or special treat, but a steady presence.

But for most of us, life is full and fast. So, the key is to start small, start simple, and start now.

It doesn't have to be perfect. It just has to begin.

Daily Nature Touchpoints (Even in a City)

Nature does not have to be far away. It can be woven into ordinary moments. Here are gentle, practical ways to invite it in:

- **Open a window and listen**: Morning birdsong, evening crickets, wind through branches. Let nature be your background soundtrack.
- **Green your commute**: Walk or bike when possible. Choosing routes with trees or water—even a few extra minutes can make a difference.
- **Create a ritual**: Drink your coffee outside. Stretch on the porch. Step outside after work and just breathe.
- **Visit the same spot often**: A bench in a park. A quiet corner near a tree. Watch how it changes over days and seasons. Let it become familiar.
- **Touch the earth**: Garden if you can. If not, water a plant, dig your hands in the soil, or rest your palms on the trunk of a tree.
- **Use your lunch break**: Even 10 minutes outside—away from screens—can reset your energy.
- **Watch the sky**: Sunrise, sunset, drifting clouds. The sky is an open canvas of nature, and it is always

there, waiting.

Weekly Deepening: Make It a Ritual, not a Task

Think of your weekly nature time as a gentle commitment to your well-being.

- Take a weekend walk in a park, along a beach, or along a forested path. Let your feet lead without rushing.
- Explore a new trail, garden, or outdoor museum. Curiosity is its own medicine. Visit water if you can—rivers, lakes, or even fountains have a calming presence. The rhythm of water has been shown to soothe the brain and regulate emotions.
- Go phone-free for a portion of your outing. Let your senses lead instead of your camera.

This isn't about adding more to your to-do list. This is about reclaiming time that restores you. Time that feels like yours.

You do not have to do it all. You just need to do something consistently.

Over time, these rituals will begin to shape you from the inside out.

For Those with Limited Access to Nature

If you are in an environment with limited greenery or mobility, you can still bring nature to you:

- **Houseplants**: Even a single plant can shift the mood of a room. Caring for it is a simple, tangible act of reciprocity.
- **Nature sounds**: Play recordings of rain, waves, or forest ambiance during your day. Studies show this can lower blood pressure and increase focus.

- **Nature visuals:** Use nature-themed screensavers or prints in your space. Looking at images of natural environments has measurable calming effects.
- **Aroma and texture:** Use essential oils (like pine or citrus), natural materials, or fresh flowers to engage the senses. Smell and touch are powerful pathways to presence.

Connection does not have to be grand to be real.

Even a moment—a beautiful leaf catching the light, a breeze through the window—can remind you that you are not separate from nature. You are part of it.

Design It Your Way

There is no perfect routine. This is not about pressure. It is about presence.

Ask yourself:

- *What kind of nature makes me feel calmer?*
- *When in my day do I feel most disconnected?*
- *Where can I trade 10 minutes of scrolling for 10 minutes outside?*

You do not need to overhaul your schedule. You simply need to shape small spaces that remind you of what matters. Build your routine like you would build a path—step by step, and with care.

Your routine is yours to shape. Start where you are. Use what you have. Go as slowly as you need.

Let it feel natural—not forced. Let it feel like you.

Closing Reflection

Nature does not ask you to be anything other than who you are.

It does not rush. It does not judge. It simply offers you a place to return to.

So, make space for it—not just on weekends or vacations, but in the small folds of your daily life.

Let it be your pause.

Your reset.

Your quiet exhale between everything else.

Because when you design time for nature, you are really designing space for yourself.

And you, too, deserve a place to soften. To slow down. To belong.

Chapter 8: Movement in Nature — Reconnecting Through the Body

There is a certain kind of freedom that only shows up when we move our bodies outdoors. Not on treadmills or under fluorescent lights, but out where the trail bends, where the ground is not flat, where the air shifts and carries the scent of pine, salt, or soil. Where movement feels less like exercise, and more like returning to the way we were meant to move—with purpose, rhythm, and breath.

This chapter explores the power of moving in nature, not just to stay fit, but to feel whole— to move through stress, return to presence, and reconnect with what it means to be alive in a body that is meant to explore the earth.

Nature-Based Exercise: Moving Beyond the Gym

There is nothing wrong with gyms. They are efficient. Structured. Controlled. But that is exactly the thing—they are controlled environments. Predictable, repetitive, closed off from the wind, the light, the texture of the world outside.

Nature-based movement—whether it is a slow walk in the woods, a hike up a trail, paddling a kayak, or climbing over rocks—engages the body in a fuller way. You are not just working muscles. You are adjusting to uneven terrain, watching light shifts, listening to sounds, breathing fresh air, feeling your body respond to the land beneath you.

You are not just exercising. You are participating—in the weather, the moment, the landscape.

The Benefits Beyond the Physical

When we move through nature, the body and mind shift together. Here is what happens:

- Stress melts gently, not in a burst of adrenaline but in a slow unraveling. The mind gets quieter with every step.
- Mood lifts naturally. The combination of movement and scenery increases endorphins and decreases tension.
- Balance and coordination improve because the terrain is varied and real—roots, rocks, slopes, inclines. Your body learns to adapt again.
- Creativity wakes up. Many people report their best ideas arriving on walks, hikes, or paddles—moments when the mind is moving but not forcing.
- Presence deepens. You become more aware of your surroundings, how the wind brushes your skin, the crunch of leaves underfoot, the sound of your own breath.
- You sleep better. A day spent moving outdoors helps reset your body clock and promotes deeper, more restful sleep.

Most importantly, you begin to trust your body again—not for how it looks or performs, but for how it carries you through the world.

Nature Does not Measure–It Meets You Where You Are

Unlike gym culture, which can sometimes focus on numbers, tracking, performance, or comparison, movement in nature has no scoreboard.

There is no perfect pace. No leaderboard. No mirrors. There is only you and the path ahead, however long, or short it may be.

Some days, it is a slow stroll in the park. Other days, it is a long hike or a climb that pushes your edges. Every day, it counts.

Ideas for Outdoor Movement (No Experience Needed)

You do not have to be a seasoned hiker or athlete to begin. Start simple:

- Take a walk after meals—let digestion and reflection happen together.
- Stretch barefoot in the grass—reconnect with the ground, breathe deeper.
- Go explore—a new trail, a nearby river path, or a community garden.
- Join a nature-based movement group—yoga in the park, walking clubs, or paddle meetups.
- Use the seasons as inspiration—snowshoe in winter, bike in spring, wade in summer, wander in fall.

Let movement outdoors be less about calories and more about connection—to yourself, to the earth, to the present moment.

Nature-Based Exercise Routines

If you are looking to bring more structure to your outdoor movement, try incorporating simple routines that connect body and breath with the natural world:

1. **Sunrise Yoga Sequence**

- Choose a quiet outdoor space.

- Begin with grounding: stand barefoot and take five slow breaths.
- Flow through a gentle sun salutation series.
- Finish seated, facing east, with hands placed at the heart.

2. **Nature Tai Chi Practice**

- Find a peaceful spot, like near a tree or flowing stream.
- Focus on slow, intentional movements that mirror water, wind, or rooted trees.
- Let your breath lead and allow pauses for stillness and presence.

3. **Walking Meditation**

- Choose a short trail or park loop.
- Walk slowly, in silence, matching your breath to your pace.
- Notice the details: textures underfoot, temperature, sounds.

4. **Wild Card Circuit**

- Pick five natural elements around you (e.g., tree, bench, hill, log, boulder).
- Do 1-minute bodyweight movements at each: squats, planks, step-ups, etc.
- Pause between deep breaths and observation.

5. **Mindful Hike & Journal**

- Take a moderate hike alone.
- Bring a small notebook.
- Pause halfway to sit, breathe, and write what you see,

feel, and think.

These routines are not about perfection, they are about presence. About remembering that your body is not separate from the natural world.

It was made to move within it.

Closing Reflection

Your body is not a machine to fine-tune. It is a living, breathing part of nature—designed to move with the wind, stretch toward the sun, and carry you through the beauty of this world.

So, walk.

Climb.

Paddle.

Wander.

Dance beneath the trees if you feel like it.

Let movement be more than exercise. Let it be a conversation between your breath and the sky. Let it be an offering to the land beneath your feet. Let it be an act of returning—to your strength, to your joy, to the rhythm of a world that was never meant to be measured in steps or reps.

Some days it may look like stillness, a pause beside a river. Other days it may be a wild run through rain or laughter on a trail.

However, it comes, let it be yours.

Unscripted. Unscored. Unashamed.

Because this body of yours is not separate from the earth. It is part of the wild. And it reminds you how to move.

Chapter 9: Green in the Gray

Finding Nature in Cities: Nature doesn't live only in forests and fields.

It grows between sidewalk cracks.

It reaches from balconies.

It surprises you in tiny corners of a concrete world—green, alive, quietly offering breath to the busy.

This chapter is about the hidden power of urban nature, the ways we find beauty, calm, and connection even in places built of steel and stone. Because even in cities, nature is not absent. It is waiting to be noticed.

Urban Nature's Hidden Power

You might not wake up to the mountains or walk past lakes on your way to work, but that does not mean nature is not near. Cities hold their own kind of wilderness, smaller, scrappier, but no less sacred.

These pockets of green may not stretch for miles, but they can still stretch your spirit. They offer moments of stillness, breath, and beauty in the middle of your daily rush. And sometimes, it is those tiny moments that make the biggest difference.

Pocket Parks and Street Trees: Little Oases of Calm

Have you ever sat in a city park and noticed how the noise seems to fade, even just a little? How does the air feel under a tree, or how your breath slows while watching leaves sway?

Pocket parks, community gardens, and street trees are not just decorative. They are essential. Research shows that even small green spaces in urban areas:

- Reduce stress and improve mood.
- Encourage walking, movement, and community connection.
- Lower urban temperatures and improve air quality.
- Help people feel more grounded and less overwhelmed.

They offer a place to pause between errands. A place to walk after dinner. A space to just *sit and not perform.*

Rooftop Gardens & Balconies: Growing Peace Over Pavement Up above the rush, something beautiful is growing.

Rooftop gardens, terraces, and balcony pots bring nature to unexpected places—above the horns, above the rush, closer to the sky. Whether it is a community food garden or a single flower box outside your apartment window, these elevated green spaces create a sense of expansion. You step outside, and suddenly, the world feels bigger again.

There is something healing about tending to a plant where none should grow. It reminds us that nature *will* find a way—and so we can.

The Power of Houseplants: Nature on Your Windowsill If you cannot go outside, bring a little outside in.

Houseplants are more than trendy, they are living reminders of nature's calm, right inside your home. They clean the air, soften your space, and provide quiet companionship.

And they require just enough care to remind you to slow down.

Watering a plant. Turning it toward the sun. Watching new leaves unfurl. These acts, though small, reconnect you with life's gentler rhythms.

Even one plant in your space can shift the energy.

A green reminder: you are not separate from the living

world—you are part of it.

Simple Ways to Find or Create Nature in the City

- Sit under a tree during your lunch break, even if it is near traffic.
- Choose the scenic route—walk past flowers, trees, or murals of natural scenes.
- Visit your local botanical garden, nature center, or urban farm.
- Place plants by windows, hang them from ceilings, or build a tiny indoor herb garden.
- Attend a community clean-up or garden planting event—connect with nature and your neighbors.
- Look up—sunsets, cloud patterns, and moonlight still visit the city.

Why It Matters

You do not need endless acres to feel nature's effect. You just need access—and attention.

In cities, nature shows up in small, defiant ways. A single flower blooming through cement. A crow calling from a rooftop. A splash of ivy climbing brick. A tree's silhouette holding the sky between buildings.

These are not accidents. They are invitations.

Closing Reflection

Even in the most crowded cities, the earth speaks—softly, persistently, through every root, leaf, and feathered wing.

So, look for it.

Look for the tree that shades your bus stop.

The fern in your bathroom.

The rooftop vines.

The flower box you pass every day but never noticed.

Because nature does not wait for the perfect setting. It simply grows where it can—and so can you.

Restoration does not always require escape. Sometimes, it begins with paying attention. Sometimes, it starts by letting the world remind you: you are not alone. You are part of this living, breathing rhythm too. And every step, every breath, every moment spent in nature is a way back home to yourself.

Chapter 10:
Seasonal Healing

Nature does not rush.

It moves in cycles and flows, bloom and rest, dark and light.

And when we begin to live in rhythm with the seasons, instead of fighting them, something in us softens. We begin to heal—not just through nature, but **with it.**

This chapter explores the power of **seasonal healing**—how each part of the year brings its own kind of wisdom, rest, and renewal. The goal is not to push against the seasons, but to **embrace their lessons**—to move with their energy, let them shape our routines, and honor the deep medicine they each offer.

Embracing Seasonality: The Nature of Change

Modern life often asks us to be the same person all year long—equally productive in July as in January, equally social in spring as in autumn. But that is not how nature works. Trees do not bloom in winter. Flowers do not rush their petals. Everything has a season—and so do we.

When we learn to live coordinated with nature's rhythm, our bodies and minds find a gentler pace. We move from exhaustion to balance. From resisting change to welcoming it.

Let us walk through the seasons, each one a teacher, each one a healer in its own way.

Spring: Energy, Awakening, and New Growth

Spring arrives like a breath after holding it too long.

It brings a sense of motion—buds swelling, rivers thawing, birds returning. In the body, this season stirs energy, possibility, and a longing to begin again.

Spring invites you to:

- Start fresh habits or revisit old ones with new softness.
- Walk outdoors and notice the first flowers, first warm breeze, first sunrise you catch without a coat.
- Plant something—even if it is just intention.
- Shake off winter's stillness through light movement, play, or creativity.

Spring reminds us that growth can be joyful, that beginnings do not have to be perfect to be beautiful.

Summer: Vitality, Expansion, and Light

Summer is full—of sound, warmth, color, and life. Days are long. The world feels open and alive.

It is a time for connection, adventure, and **staying out a little longer**—with people, with places, with the sky.

Summer invites you to:

- Move your body in big, open ways, hike, dance, wander.
- Spend more time barefoot, sun-kissed, and unhurried.
- Soak in the light—not just with your skin, but with your spirit.
- Celebrate what is in bloom—around you, and within you.

Summer teaches us to *expand without apology*, to gather joy like sun on the skin.

Autumn: Reflection, Release, and Rebalancing Autumn is the season of turning inward.

The days begin to contract. The trees let go. The air cools, and with it comes a quiet invitation to pause—to reflect, to harvest, and to release what is no longer needed.

Autumn invites you to:

- Let go of what you have outgrown—habits, expectations, even clutter.
- Reassess your pace, your goals, your inner balance.
- Walk among the falling leaves and ask yourself: What am I ready to set down?
- Create warmth indoors—through journaling, candlelight, nourishing food.

Autumn reminds us that **letting go is not a loss, it is preparation**. It is the way we make space for what matters.

Winter: Stillness, Rest, and Deep Restoration

Winter is the great exhale. The retreat inward. The blanket pulled over tired bones.

It is the season most often resisted—and yet, it offers the deepest healing if we let it. Beneath the quiet is a richness: the rest that precedes all growth, the pause that allows everything else to unfold.

Winter invites you to:

- Slow down your schedule and listen to your natural rhythms.
- Rest more—not as laziness, but as intentional renewal.
- Light fires (real or symbolic) and gather warmth.
- Reflect—not to plan, but simply to be in the moment.

Winter teaches us the **power of stillness**, and the sacredness of not producing, not pushing, just being.

Living in Rhythm

We were not meant to live in a constant state of output.

We were not designed to bloom all year round, to stay energized in the dead of winter, or to feel the same every day of the year. But modern life has taught us to ignore these natural shifts—to override the seasons in our bodies, our minds, our emotions.

And yet, the earth keeps reminding us: there is time for everything.

When we begin to align ourselves with the seasons—not perfectly, but intentionally—we reconnect with a quieter truth. We remember that ebb is just as important as flow, that slowness is not failure, and that rest is not the opposite of growth, it is a part of it.

Each season offers a different kind of medicine:

- Spring brings possibility and newness, reminding us it is safe to start again.
- Summer encourages us to open up, to say yes, to stretch toward joy.
- Autumn helps us release, reassess, and clear space for what matters.
- Winter invites us to soften, to listen inward, and to restore without guilt.

When we pay attention to these rhythms, we notice similar cycles within ourselves: times of energy and action, times of reflection and retreat. We move through the year with more awareness, more compassion, and more grace.

It is not about doing more.

It is about doing differently choosing to act in ways that support the season you are in, both outside and within.

You are allowed to shift.

To rest. To grow slowly. To feel different in July than you do in January.

You are allowed to be cyclical, emotional, uncertain, and vibrant—all in turn.

You are not separate from the seasons. You are made of them.

So let the rhythm of the earth be your guide—not as a schedule to follow, but as a permission slip to live more fully, more freely, and more in tune with your own becoming.

Closing Reflection

Let the seasons set your rhythm.

Let Spring awaken what is been sleeping.

Let summer stretch you toward the light.

Let autumn guide you into the art of release. Let winter wrap you in rest without guilt.

Because healing is not linear.

It moves in cycles—in soft returns, in quiet shifts. It spirals, deepens, and begins again.

And nature will be there—patient, steady—at every turn.

Chapter 11: Your 30-Day Nature Reset

You do not need to escape your life to reconnect with nature.

You do not need a sabbatical or a remote cabin.

You just need **a moment**—a breath, a pause, a patch of sky—and the willingness to begin.

This chapter is your invitation to gently **reweave nature back into your days**. Not as another task on a to-do list, but as a way of returning to yourself. One small, meaningful step at a time.

Over the next 30 days, you will find simple practices designed to help you slow down, restore focus, and reconnect with the world around you—even in the middle of a busy, urban, tech-filled life. Most activities take less than 15 minutes, and you can adapt them to suit your schedule, energy, and environment.

This reset is not about perfection. It is about presence. Let it be soft. Let it be yours.

Your 30-Day Nature Reset: Daily Practices for Reconnection

A month of mindful reconnection, one day at a time. Each invitation below is a gentle opening—to breath, to beauty, to presence.

Day 1: Step outside first thing in the morning.

Before you check your phone or look at a screen, open your door and step out. Feel the air on your skin. Hear the earliest sounds of life beginning again. Let the world greet you.

Day 2: Take a 10-minute mindful walk.

Choose a short route. Walk without rushing. Let your attention land on colors, textures, shadows, and smells. Be curious. Be slow.

Day 3: Bring a houseplant into your space.

Choose one that feels inviting. Give it a name if you like. Let its quiet growth remind you that life is always unfolding, even when it moves slowly.

Day 4: Watch the sky for five full minutes.

Find a place to sit or lie down. Watch without expectation. Notice cloud shapes, light movement, or the stillness of blue. Let it shift something inside you.

Day 5: Journal outside, even if it is just a few lines.

Bring a notebook or piece of paper. Write what you see. What you hear. What does your body feel. No edits. Just observation.

Day 6: Sit beneath a tree.

Let the shade hold you. Listen to the leaves. Feel how steady and grounded it is. Let some of that steadiness become yours.

Day 7: Eat one meal outdoors.

It can be as simple as a snack on the porch. Notice how the wind feels, how flavors shift, how your body responds when you are surrounded by sky.

Day 8: Collect a small object from nature.

A stone, a shell, a feather. Let it rest somewhere visible. Let it anchor your day.

Day 9: Open a window.

Just for a moment, let the breeze in. Listen. Smell. Feel the difference fresh air makes.

Day 10: Walk a different route today.

Break your routine. Choose the more scenic option. Let your senses lead. Let the unfamiliar awaken your attention.

Day 11: Sketch something from nature.

Even if you have not drawn in years, try. Follow the lines of a leaf. Capture the curve of a flower. Let yourself see more by slowing down.

Day 12: Listen to nature sounds before bed.

Choose a soundscape—rain, forest, ocean—and play it softly. Let it be your lullaby.

Day 13: Spend five minutes barefoot on grass or earth.

Let the soles of your feet touch the ground. Wiggle your toes. Feel supported.

Day 14: Visit a nearby park or green space.

Sit with no goal. Let nature do the talking. Let your nervous system settle.

Day 15: Tend to a plant.

Give it water. Trim the dead leaves. Speak to it if you want. Let it remind you of growth without pressure.

Day 16: Watch a sunrise or sunset.

Make space for the shift in light. Let it soften your thoughts. Let it close or open your day with reverence.

Day 17: Pick up a piece of litter on your walk.

Do it not out of guilt, but care. A quiet gesture of reciprocity.

Day 18: Write a short nature poem.

Let it be playful or tender or raw. Let it capture one single moment. Four lines. One breath.

Day 19: Sit outside in silence for 10 minutes.

Do not fill the time. Let the silence stretch. Let it reveal what is been underneath the noise.

Day 20: Look up at the stars.

Feel how small and held you are. Let awe rise in your chest. Let it remind you that you belong.

Day 21: Place fresh flowers or greenery in your home.

Let color brighten your space. Let life live where you are.

Day 22: Take a walk in the rain (or imagine it).

Let yourself be part of the weather. Feel each drop. Let discomfort become presence.

Day 23: Create a tiny altar of natural things.

Arrange a small space with leaves, stones, feathers, whatever feels sacred. Visit it when you need grounding.

Day 24: Sit with a tree and imagine its life.

What storms has it weathered? What seasons has it seen? Let its rootedness speak to your own.

Day 25: Lay on the ground and look up.

Let gravity hold your body. Let the sky remind you how vast it is to be alive.

Day 26: Write about a memory in nature that brought you peace. Close your eyes. Return there. Describe every detail. Feel it again.

Day 27: Try a nature-based meditation.

Visualize roots growing from your feet. Imagine yourself as a mountain, a stream, a tree. Let nature live inside you.

Day 28: Light a candle or lantern as the sun sets.

Mark the change. Let it be a gentle pause. A soft moment of transition.

Day 29: Visit water—any kind.

Let it reflect you. Let it remind you to move, to flow, to release.

Day 30: Reflect on what changed.

Write or speak aloud: What softened? What surprised you? What do you want to carry into tomorrow?

Closing Reflection: Carrying Nature with You

By now, you may have realized: this was not about adding something new. It was about remembering what has always been there—the sky above you, the ground beneath you, the quiet call to come home to the present.

Let this reset be a beginning, not an end. Keep walking slowly. Keep watching leaves. Keep finding wonder in small things.

Because you are not separate from nature. You are part of its rhythm, its story, its unfolding. And it will always be there, ready to welcome you back.

Chapter 12:
Let the Water Speak

Some truths do not arrive as answers.

They arrive as ripples—small, steady movements that travel through us long after the surface has calmed.

This chapter is not about knowing. It is about listening.

Because water has a way of holding space for the things we have not put into words yet.

The things we carry quietly. The things we try to tidy away.

Water does not rush us to clarity. It does not push for perfection. It simply receives.

Begin with Stillness

Find a quiet place—ideally near real water. A pond, a stream, a fountain. If that is not possible, let memory or imagination guide you. A bathtub. A window with rain. A sound recording of waves. A photo of a lake you once loved.

Find a quiet location where you can sit comfortably and without distractions. Allow your body to settle into the chair beneath you. Relax your shoulders, unclench your jaw, and release any tension in your hands. Permit gravity to support you, and let the ground hold you securely.

Close your eyes. Inhale slowly, as if drawing in the air deliberately. Exhale with even greater control, as if releasing an unnecessary thought.

Repeat this process. Continue to do so. Each breath serves as a gentle recalibration.

Now, begin to imagine the presence of water.

See it in your mind's eye:

A still pond, its surface dappled with sunlight.

A gentle river, weaving over smooth stones.

The rhythmic pull and release of waves folding into the shore.

Notice the movement—unhurried, continuous, alive.

Feel how it has no destination, no urgency. It simply flows.

And with every breath, let your body mirror that motion.

Let your inhale rise like a wave.

Let your exhale fall like the tide.

Let your mind quiet, not by force, but by following the natural rhythm of water.

Feel its calm settle into you—cool, fluid, grounding.

Let it wash through the places that feel tight or tired.

Let it gather the things you have been carrying and begin to soften their edges.

There is no right way to do this.

There is only presence. Only breath. Only the flow of this moment.

Let the water guide you. Let it hold you.

Let it remind you what it feels like to **be at ease within yourself.**

Let the Questions Come

When you feel calm, open—not to productivity, but to presence—ask yourself gently:

- *What am I carrying that feels heavy right now?*
- *What am I ready to release, even if I do not fully understand it yet?*

- *If water could speak to me today, what would it say?*

Do not chase the answers. Let them come to you, like driftwood floating toward the shore.

Now, begin to write.

Not carefully. Not perfectly. Not with the intention to be understood.

Let this be a release, not a performance. Longhand, if you can—pen to paper, slow and real. There is something grounding in the physical act of writing, something ancient and honest that typing cannot always reach.

Do not worry about punctuation or grammar or whether your words fit together like puzzle pieces.

Let them drift. Let them collide. Let them contradict.

You are not writing for clarity—you are writing for movement.

Let the words spill out the way water does—without apology, without resistance. Let the thoughts rise like waves and break as they will. Some may make sense. Others may not.

You may find yourself writing the same phrase three times. You may drift into memory, into wish, into ache. That is okay.

You are not writing a story.

You are not solving a problem. You are making space.

You are catching fragments—flashes of emotion, images that will not leave you, things your body knows but your mind has not named. You are writing from the part of you that does not speak in tidy paragraphs, but in feelings, in rhythms, in currents.

This is not for anyone else to read. This is for you.

The self beneath the surface. The voice that often goes unheard. The truths that do not arrive in full sentences, but in sensations.

Write as if water were listening—because in a way, it is.

It listens the way only nature does: without judgment, without interruption, without needing you to explain.

Let this be your offering to the page. Let it be messy, tender, unfinished. Let it be true. And if nothing comes, write that too.

I do not know what I am feeling. I do not know where to begin. But I am here.

Sometimes, presence is more powerful than precision. Sometimes, writing is not a record, it is a release.

Let it be what it is. Let it flow.

Why It Heals

This kind of journaling is not about solving problems.

It is about **creating a safe container** for what is inside to move.

When we write beside (or within) the energy of water, something unspoken often surfaces.

A long-held fear. An old memory. A desire we have not made room for. Often, it arrives subtly—not to overpower, but to be observed.

Water, in its way, makes it okay to feel without needing to explain.

To let things move without fixing them.

To let go, without knowing where they will land.

If Water Could Speak...

What would it say?

Would it whisper: *You do not have to carry this alone*?

Would it hum: *Even this will pass*?

Would it remind you: *You are not stuck, you are flowing, always*?

Whatever you imagine what it might say, let that be your message.

Write it down. Return to it.

Make it your anchor when you forget how to breathe.

Closing Practice

When your writing feels complete, read it softly—just to yourself.

Then close your journal and place your hand over your heart.

Take one more breath and imagine that your words have been offered to the water—not to disappear, but to be transformed.

Because this is what water does.

It receives. It moves.

It reshapes the hard edges.

And if you let it, so will you.

Chapter 13: Earthing—Remembering with Your Feet

Take off your shoes. Stand on the ground—just as you are. Barefoot. Simple. Direct.

Let your feet contact the real surface beneath you—grass, soil, stone, sand, or even warm pavement. Wiggle your toes. Feel the temperature, the texture, the unevenness. It may feel unfamiliar at first, especially if you haven't done it in a while. But soon, your body begins to remember.

We spend most of our lives separated from the earth by layers—of rubber soles, concrete, flooring. We rush from place to place, rarely pausing to notice what's beneath us. But our bodies were built to connect with the ground. To feel it directly. To calibrate to its steadiness.

Walking barefoot—sometimes called *earthing*—isn't about following a trend. It's about returning to something simple and real. When your skin touches the ground, your attention shifts. You slow down. You breathe differently. You come back to yourself.

Even just a few steps barefoot outdoors can activate something physical and emotional. It regulates the nervous system. It helps the body settle. It reminds you that you're supported, literally, from the ground up.

And sometimes, that connection happens when you least expect it.

An Unexpected Moment: Barefoot in Costa Rica

I was on a guided walk through the rainforest in Costa Rica

when we reached a shallow lake we needed to cross. I quickly removed my shoes and waded in, thinking I'd stop switching into water shoes on the other side. But the guide spotted signs of nearby animal activity and urged me to keep moving.

There wasn't time to pause. So, I kept going—barefoot.

At first, I was uneasy. The ground was muddy, uneven, full of unfamiliar textures. My focus was on every step: what I might be stepping on, where my balance was, how far I had to go. But after a few minutes, something shifted. The nervousness gave way to awareness.

I noticed the way the earth felt underfoot—cool, textured, alive. The sensation of walking barefoot through the rainforest wasn't just physical, it was a full-body kind of presence. There were no distractions. Just the trail, the sounds of the forest, the focused calm of our guide ahead, and my feet meeting the world with every step.

And to my surprise, it wasn't just bearable, it was exhilarating.

Without shoes, I wasn't removed from the place—I was *in it.* Every step brought me deeper into the experience, not just of movement, but of belonging. I felt more awake, more connected, more human.

That moment reminded me that sometimes grounding doesn't come through stillness. It comes through unexpected challenges. Through discomfort that leads to awareness. Through a moment when everything else fades away and you remember what it means to truly *feel* the earth beneath you.

Reconnection, One Step at a Time

We don't have to wait for perfect conditions to reconnect.

We don't need a forest trail or a guided experience.

You can step into your own yard. A beach. A trail. Even a patch of grass outside your door.

Start small.

Take off your shoes.

Stand still. Notice.

You may find your thoughts slow down. Your shoulders are dropping. Your breath deepening. There's something very steady about standing barefoot on the earth. The world doesn't ask anything of you at that moment. It just holds you.

Shoes, schedules, and screens often shield us from discomfort—but they also shield us from connection. Earthing removes a barrier. And what it offers in return is presence. Clarity. Calm.

Closing Reflection

You don't need a perfect place to begin.

You don't need to know exactly what you're looking for.

You just need a patch of ground—and the willingness to pause.

Let your feet meet the earth.

Let your breath catch up to you.

Let your body remember what it's like to simply *be*.

This is not about doing something right.

It's about being somewhere real.

And in that reality, you may find something you didn't even know you were missing.

The earth doesn't care about your to-do list.

It doesn't ask for performance. It only asks for presence.

So, take off your shoes.

Arrive fully.

And let the ground welcome you home.

Chapter 14: The Park Bench Pause

Walk without a goal.

Sit without a plan.

Let the birdsong fill your ears. Let the breeze press gently against your skin. Notice how your breath begins to shift—how your shoulders lower, how the edges of your thoughts soften.

You do not have to solve anything here.

You do not have to perform.

You are allowed to simply be.

The bench is more than a place to rest tired legs.

It is an altar of stillness.

A threshold into presence.

It does not ask anything of you except that you *stop moving.* That you *witness* the world as it is—without the need to change it, fix it, or control it.

The Sacred Ordinary

I've spent many afternoons doing nothing but sitting. Letting the light shift through branches, counting squirrels as they leap from trunk to trunk, listening to conversations I'll never be a part of but somehow feel comforted by. Footsteps, bicycle bells, someone humming off-key.

There's a quiet intimacy in being part of the background.

In that stillness, everything starts to feel more alive: The glint of sunlight on the park pond.

The rustle of leaves shifting direction with the wind.

The laughter of a child weaving in and out of playground noise. A couple walking past, lost in quiet conversation.

It's not dramatic. It's not curated.

And maybe that's the whole point.

There's something healing about witnessing the unremarkable. The way time slows down when you're not trying to shape it into something else. The way meaning emerges when you stop reaching for it.

A Place Without Pressure

There is no agenda on a bench.

No metrics to meet.

No pressure to be productive.

Just a permission slip for stillness.

And sometimes, when you stop striving, life begins to show itself again. A bird might land close enough for you to hear the rustle of its feathers. The breeze might rearrange the leaves in a way that catches your attention for no reason at all. The sun might strike a spider web just right, turning it to lace.

These are not grand revelations.

They are quiet reminders:

You are still part of the world.

You are still being met by wonder.

And you don't have to chase it.

Let Nature Do the Talking

There is a special kind of listening that happens when you stop talking. When you stop moving. When you allow the world to arrive as it is, without your interference.

Let the wind speak in the language of rustling trees.

Let the birds carry the melody of the moment.

Let your nervous system remember what calm feels like—not in theory, but in the lived rhythm of your breath syncing with the pace of the earth.

When you sit without intention, you make space.

And in that space, presence finds its way back to you.

When Doing Nothing Becomes Everything

We are so accustomed to measuring our worth by what we *do*, tasks completed, boxes checked, goals pursued—that we forget something essential:

The body longs to pause.

The spirit, too, needs room to stretch without striving.

In a world that glorifies motion, stillness becomes a radical act.

We think we must keep moving to grow, but not everything grows in sunlight. Some things deepen in the dark. Some things blossom only when we stop tending to outcomes and start tending to presence.

The breath deepens not through force, but through permission.

The heart opens not through willpower, but through quiet.

And some of the most meaningful moments in life don't arrive with noise and drama— they emerge in the pause between things.

In the silence after a long thought.

In the way your shoulders drop when no one is watching. In the simple relief of *not needing to be anywhere else.*

Stillness does not mean disengaged.

It means rooted.

It means aware.

It means choosing not to rush because this moment—right here—already holds enough.

It is the art of presence.

The practice of letting the world arrive on its own terms.

When you sit without expectation, the sky begins to speak again.

Not with answers, but with light shifting on leaves.

With the hum of bees.

With the hush of breeze against your cheek.

You are not wasting time on a bench.

You are reclaiming it.

You are remembering that you are not a machine, but a human—meant to rest, to breathe, to feel the sun on your skin without explanation.

Doing nothing, in truth, is not doing *nothing* at all.

It is listening.

It is softening.

It is returning to the rhythm that life itself has always kept.

And in that return, something forgotten within you starts to bloom.

Closing Reflection

You do not need to go far to return to yourself.

Sometimes, a single bench beneath a tree is enough.

Let the world move around you while you stay still.

Let the air settle.

Let your heartbeat slow.

This moment asks nothing of you.

You do not need to make sense of anything.

You do not need to fix or change. You are allowed to just *be.*

Sit.

Notice the light.

Listen to the breeze.

Let the birds do the speaking.

Because when you stop running toward meaning, sometimes it finds you anyway.

Stillness is not an absence.

It is a doorway.

And the park bench, humble and quiet, may just be the place where you walk through.

Chapter 15: The Nature of Sleep

Rest is a birthright, yet modern life often steals it from us.

We stay up too late under fluorescent light, overstimulated by screens that never dim, filling our minds with noise long after the sun has gone quiet. We wake to alarms instead of rhythms, push through fatigue as though tiredness is a flaw, and fill our days until there's no space left to unwind.

But sleep, at its core, is not a weakness or an afterthought—it is a rhythm. A natural, ancient rhythm that the body has always known and that the earth still remembers.

When we begin to live more in step with the world outside—exposing our eyes to morning light, spending more time under open skies, honoring dusk instead of resisting it—something inside us recalibrates. Our bodies start to remember the old cues. The ones that existed before schedules and screens. Before caffeine and calendars. The ones that lived in light and shadow, in temperature and sound.

Sunlight in the morning resets our internal clock, signaling to the brain: *Now is the time to wake.* But equally powerful is the softening of light at day's end, the way the shadows stretch across the ground, the way the wind cools, the way everything, even the noise of the day, begins to quiet. Dusk is nature's lullaby. And if we listen, it begins to soften us too.

Even ten minutes outside in the fading light can downshift the nervous system. It slows the heartbeat.

It lowers the pulse.

It whispers: *You can stop now. You've done enough.*

The Companionship of Night

There is something sacred about an open window at night. The air flows carrying the scent of damp soil, the pulse of cool wind, the steady murmur of the world continuing on without urgency. You hear the hush of leaves brushing against one another. The bark of a distant dog. The rhythmic chorus of crickets or frogs composing a kind of nocturnal prayer.

This is not silence. This is symphony.

And your body listens.

Your breath begins to match the rhythm outside. Your heart slows. The tension held in the shoulders, the jaw, the gut—begins to dissolve, almost without notice. Sleep doesn't come crashing in. It arrives the way fog rolls over the hills—softly, completely, without needing to announce itself.

Even darkness, when experienced this way, feels different. Not empty, not frightening—but alive. Held. Cradled. Less like an absence of light and more like an invitation to go inward.

This is what the natural world offers:

Not just quiet, but kinship. Not just rest, but return.

The Deep Rest of Wildness

Some people rediscover this rhythm by sleeping outside, if only for a night or two. A tent beneath the stars. A cabin without curtains. A hammock under branches that moves with the wind. And in those nights—when no devices hum and no clocks glow—they find something they didn't know were missing true, unfiltered rest.

To sleep beneath the stars is to let the earth hold you.

To surrender the body to temperature, to sound, to stillness.

To let your breath match the breeze, your heartbeat aligns with the rustle of the trees.

Out there, there are no deadlines.

Only the slow, steady passage of time marked by moonrise and birdcall.

You fall asleep to the sounds of owls or wind or the shifting of leaves.

And you wake with the first light—soft and gold, not blaring. A reminder that you, too, are part of a cycle.

And in this rhythm, something inside you reawakens.

Not because you forced it.

But because you finally stopped forcing everything else.

Because rest does not come when we've earned it—it comes when we *allow* it. And the earth, patient as ever, is always offering the cue.

Letting Rest Be Enough

There is a kind of rest that no supplement or sleep aid can provide. The kind that comes not from exhaustion, but from alignment.

When we let ourselves rest with the rhythms of the earth—rising with the light, softening with the dark—we don't just sleep.

We *belong*.

We remember that we are not machines to be optimized, but living, breathing ecosystems with needs that are more ancient than any calendar could define.

We remember that rest is not laziness, it is intelligence. It is listening. It is repair.

And most of all, it is permission.

Closing Reflection

Rest is not a luxury.

It is not something you earn.

It is a return—to self, to rhythm, to trust.

Each night, the natural world extends a quiet invitation: *You may let go now.* Let go of striving.

Let go of perfection.

Let go of the noise that insists you should always be doing more.

You do not need to wait for exhaustion to honor your need for rest. Begin small.

Take a walk in fading light.

Open the window and let the night air brush your skin.

Let the sound of leaves be your lullaby.

Let the darkness feel like comfort, not threat.

Sleep is not failure.

It is belonging.

It is your body remembering the world it came from.

And when you rest in rhythm with the earth, you are not falling behind. You are falling into place.

Chapter 16: Thresholds and Transitions

There are moments in nature that ask us to pause—not because they demand attention, but because they deserve it.

A sunrise easing its way into the sky. The moment just before the first snow falls. The last leaf clinging to a branch before drifting silently to the ground. These are not merely scenes. They are sacred thresholds—markers of passage, reminders that change is not a disruption, but a natural and necessary rhythm of life.

These transitions are gentle instructors. They do not speak in commands. They whisper: *Watch. Wait. Listen.*

The sunrise doesn't ask the sky's permission before spilling color across the horizon. It simply arrives—some days soft and pastel like a sigh, other days bold and crimson like fire. No two sunrises are ever the same, yet each carries the same truth: that light returns, and every return is slightly new. That transformation happens daily, without announcement.

A single falling leaf contains a lesson in surrender. It does not fight the wind. It trusts gravity. It floats down with grace. And in doing so, it becomes something else—soil, nourishment, part of the cycle.

Nature holds these passages with reverence. And we, too, are invited to do the same.

Holding the In-Between

In a world that often rewards hustle and productivity, it can feel unfamiliar—even uncomfortable—to honor the in-between. But nature makes no apologies for these pauses. Trees do not explain their bare branches in winter. The moon does not apologize for its dark phases. Caterpillars do not rush through the chrysalis.

Everything alive knows the value of stillness. Of gestation. Of transition.

We are not designed to stay constant. We are not meant to always bloom. We are meant to become.

And becoming takes time.

Thresholds We Often Miss

Not all transitions arrive with fanfare. Many are subtle, internal, and unspoken. The moment you realize you're ready to release a long-held resentment. The day your anxiety doesn't grip quite tightly. The quiet awareness that you're no longer in survival mode— you're beginning to feel again, to trust again, to soften.

These are thresholds too.

They may not come with ceremony or announcement, but they mark real change.

There's the edge of sleep, when thought dissolves into rest.

The first breath of a new season—the one that smells different, sharper, or warmer than yesterday.

The silence after a hard goodbye.

The pause before you tell someone the truth you've been holding inside.

These liminal spaces—the in-between moments—are not empty. They are full of movement, full of meaning. They hold both past and possibility at once. Like the twilight between night and day, they are places where who you've been and who you're becoming briefly overlap.

And yet, we often rush through them.

Distracted. Preoccupied. Focused on the next thing.

But when we slow down long enough to notice these moments—when we mark them in even the smallest ways—

we create space for something deeper.

Lighting a candle at dusk.

Sitting quietly before beginning something new.

Taking a longer breath before replying.

Walking slowly through change instead of rushing to the next chapter.

These simple acts aren't about rituals for ritual's sake. They're about presence. About meeting ourselves inside transition instead of bypassing it.

Because to recognize a threshold is to acknowledge that something is shifting.

It's to say: *I see this. I feel it. I'm here for it.*

And that awareness, however quiet, is a form of reverence.

When we honor transitions, even the subtle ones, we signal to ourselves that our experiences matter. That inner change is worth noticing. Not every chapter has to be loud to be meaningful.

Because sometimes, the smallest thresholds carry the biggest truth: You are changing.

You are moving forward.

And it's okay to take your time crossing over.

Reflection Prompt

What threshold are you standing on right now?

It may be something visible—like a career change, a move, or a new season of life. Or it may be internal slow release, a shift in perspective, a quiet beginning.

- What are you leaving behind?
- What are you beginning to move toward?

- What might help you cross this threshold with intention, instead of urgency?

Take a few moments to sit with these questions, without pressure to answer perfectly. The noticing itself is enough.

Suggested Ritual: Marking a Quiet Transition

You don't need a formal ceremony to honor change. A simple moment of intention can be powerful.

Try this:

- Choose a time of day that feels transitional—sunrise, sunset, or just before bed.
- Light a candle, step outside, or sit by a window.
- Say something quietly to yourself, like:

"Something is shifting, and I am here for it."

"I'm letting go of ____. I'm open to ____. I give myself permission to begin again."

- Breathe in. Breathe out. Let the moment be enough.

Repeat weekly, monthly, or whenever you sense something new beginning inside you.

Becoming Again and Again

Nature doesn't give us just one beginning. It gives us many, each one wrapped in a different kind of light.

Each season invites us to start again in a different way. The budding of spring does not erase the rest of the tree's life. It *builds* upon it. The shedding of autumn is not a death—it is a preparation. A clearing. A sacred exhale.

You, too, are allowed to evolve in layers.

To release.

To rise.

To return to yourself as many times as you need.

Transformation doesn't need to be dramatic or meaningful. Sometimes, it looks like resting more deeply. Saying no more clearly. Trusting joy again. Sometimes, it's a quiet decision to meet yourself with tenderness rather than critique.

Walking Through the Doorway

Life is made up of thresholds, beginnings, endings, and the blurry places in between. Some we recognize right away: weddings, births, heartbreak, moves, farewells. Others take time to name: the shift from fear to trust, from numbness to feeling, from avoidance to acceptance.

You may not always realize you've crossed into a new chapter until you look back and see how far you've come.

But nature sees you.

It honors every quiet crossing.

The sun keeps rising, even when you feel behind.

The tides keep turning, even when you stand still. The light returns in its own time, always.

Closing Reflection

Transitions are not meant to be rushed.

They are doorways—some wide, some barely cracked open. But all of them are sacred.

Let nature remind you: change can be slow.

Letting go can be gentle.

You do not need to understand it all to walk through it.

When the sky changes color, when the leaf lets go, when the light softens at the end of day—pause. Let yourself be there. Even if just for a breath. Even if it feels small.

You do not need a ceremony to begin again.

You need only awareness.

You need only the willingness to witness your own unfolding.

Because every sunset, every tide, every season turning is a reminder:

You are not stuck.

You are in motion.

You are allowed to begin again—not just once, but always.

And like the natural world around you, you are not meant to stay the same. You are meant to change, soften, strengthen, shed, and grow.

Let yourself cross the next threshold with grace.

With presence.

And with the quiet knowing that life is meeting you there.

Chapter 17: Foraging for Presence To forage is to pay attention.

It is to move slowly through the world with your senses open, your breath unhurried, and your eyes tuned not to what is obvious, but to what is quietly waiting to be seen.

Foraging is not only about gathering wild food, but also about gathering presence. It is a living conversation with the land, one built on reciprocity, observation, and humility. It teaches us that the earth gives in whispers, not shouts.

It asks us to walk without urgency. To crouch. To look under the leaves. To notice the places where life thrives low to the ground, hidden in plain sight. To ask, *what grows here?* Not just with curiosity, but with care.

There is a sacredness in this slowness. It transforms a walk into a pilgrimage.

It turns a patch of weeds into a world.

It shifts our gaze from seeking what is *useful* to appreciating what is simply *here.*

Even in most urban places—along alleyways, fence lines, and sidewalk cracks—there is something to find. A sprig of mint pushing through gravel. Wild fennel swaying beside a chain-link fence. Dandelions breaking open with gold at your feet. These are not accidents. These are reminders: the wild still finds us.

The Hidden Offerings

One spring, I wandered through a city park tracing the edges of a forgotten path. I wasn't searching for anything. I just wanted to walk slowly, without a goal, and let the land speak first.

That's when I saw them—mushrooms gathered in a quiet cluster at the base of a tree, their caps round and damp, their gills hidden like folded maps. I crouched beside them and let my eyes adjust. There were details I had never noticed before—the soft scalloped edges, the pale shifts in tone, the way their bodies rose from decaying leaves with a quiet dignity.

A shaft of sunlight slipped through the canopy, illuminating the curve of one cap from behind. Suddenly, its texture shimmered. Translucent threads glowed like veins of gold. It felt like seeing through the surface of the world into its inner workings. A private invitation. A wordless miracle.

I didn't touch them.

They weren't asking to be taken. They were asking to be seen.

And in seeing them, I noticed something else shift—inside me. My breath slowed. My thoughts quieted. My presence deepened. I was not gathering ingredients. I was gathering stillness. Reverence. A small, essential kind of awe.

The Gift of Noticing

Foraging sharpens our attention—not just to what can be harvested, but to what is offered. It asks us to pay attention to detail, to timing, to environment. But more than that, it invites a shift in mindset: from taking to relating.

The more we observe, the more we realize that not everything is meant to be gathered. Some things are there simply to be seen. Noticing becomes its own form of participation— a quiet act of respect. We stop assuming the world is here to serve us and begin to understand that we are part of a larger, living system that works whether or not we interrupt it.

Some moments aren't meant to be collected. They're meant to be honored.

Like the spiderweb I once saw suspended between two low branches, holding morning rain like pearls on silk. Each droplet refracted the light in its own direction, scattering brightness in ways no photograph could fully capture. The web shimmered like a constellation—so precise, so fragile, so alive in that brief intersection of light and water and tension. I stood there in silence, realizing that it had likely taken hours to build and would be gone by midday. Its impermanence made it more beautiful, not less.

Or the jasmine blooming outside my home one evening. I hadn't planned to stop. I was on my way inside when the scent caught me—soft, heady, almost nostalgic. It drifted through the air like something familiar I couldn't place. The white petals seemed to glow faintly in the low light, unfolding into the evening with no urgency, no need for acknowledgment. They weren't trying to be noticed. They weren't there for me. They just were.

And in that simplicity, something shifted.

Noticing isn't passive. It's relational. When we stop long enough to really see what's in front of us—whether or not we pick it, photograph it, or understand it—we start to remember how to be in the world without rushing through it.

The act of noticing is what makes the ordinary sacred. It creates a pause between what we experience and how we respond. It is where reverence begins.

In that pause, we soften.

We listen.

We let the moment be enough.

And that, too, is a kind of nourishment.

Presence as Devotion

To forage is to practice a quiet kind of faithfulness—not to the outcome, but to the moment itself.

It is to slow your pace not because you're weary, but because something inside you has finally awakened.

It is to allow wonder to disrupt your plans.

To pause mid-step because something glimmered, or grew, or called for your attention in a voice only stillness can hear.

Foraging teaches us to be moved by the small, the overlooked, the wild things growing beyond our control.

The unmarked. The uncultivated. Weeds with names we've forgotten and stories we haven't yet learned to read.

This kind of attention becomes a form of devotion.

Not the ceremonial kind—but the living kind.

The kind that arrives softly when we stop striving and ask, *what is here now, waiting to be seen?*

And in that shift, we begin to see differently.

More than that—we begin to belong differently.

The moss on stone becomes a teacher of softness.

The dandelion becomes a quiet prophet of resilience.

Even the curled decay of last season's leaves becomes sacred text.

Foraging, then, becomes less about collecting and more about returning— To attention.

To humility.

To the relationships we forgot we were part of.

You don't need to bring home anything to feel nourished.

Sometimes, the breath of jasmine in the evening, or the gleam of dew on a mushroom cap, is more than enough.

Sometimes, being with it—fully, reverently—is the harvest.

Closing Reflection

To forage is to listen with your whole body.

It is to trust that the world is still offering itself to you, even in the smallest ways.

Let the cracks in the sidewalk become invitations.

Let the wild herbs become reminders that resilience lives low to the ground. Let your steps slow—not to arrive somewhere, but to arrive *here.*

You don't need to harvest anything to feel held by the land.

You don't need to name every plant to learn from it.

You only need to be present, to be quiet, to be open.

Because what foraging truly gives us is not just flavor, not just beauty—but presence. And in presence, we remember what it feels like to be part of something—not separate from it.

This is not about taking.

It is about noticing.

It is about bowing, internally or literally, to the abundance that surrounds us.

And in that bowing, you return to something sacred.

Something simple. Something true.

So go out.

Not to collect, but to connect.

Not to gather, but to *remember.*

That even the smallest encounter—one mushroom, one

scent, one moment of stillness— can become a doorway back to wonder. And wonder, when tended, becomes a way of life.

Chapter 18: Animal Teachers

Animals do not rush.

They do not multitask.

They do not check their reflection or overthink their place in the world. They live inside instinct, rhythm, and presence.

And if we let them, they can teach us how to return to our own.

There is something grounding in watching a bird gather twigs with quiet diligence, or in the determined leap of a squirrel from branch to branch, trusting the arc of its body before its paws ever land. There is no second-guessing. No hesitation. No noise in the mind. Just motion. Just trust.

Watch a squirrel closely, and you'll see something close to reverence in its rituals—the practiced paws choosing, storing, sorting. The pause before movement. The deliberate way it holds a nut, as if nothing else matters. Even the way it locks eyes with you—curious, unafraid—feels like a reminder: *Are you paying attention? Because I am.*

Then there is the bird—gliding in slow arcs across the sky, then landing precisely where it needs to be.

No stress. No checklist. No fanfare.

Just instinct, paired with care.

A nest is not built, it is *woven.*

Layer by layer, twig by thread, shaped by breath and body. A soft architecture of safety and intention.

Animals do not force anything.

They do not question rest.

They give energy fully and then stop without apology.

A cat stretches luxuriously in a patch of sunlight and does not rush to be productive. A fox listens with stillness that is more alive than movement. A herd of elk pauses mid-meadow, scanning the horizon with calm alertness—not fear, just awareness.

In a culture that glorifies output, animals model a different kind of wisdom: To move with clarity.

To rest without guilt.

To trust the rhythm of enough.

Small Creatures, Big Lessons

Even the smallest animals carry enormous insight.

- **Bees** remind us of devotion—returning again and again to the task at hand, moving in quiet cooperation, building something greater than themselves.
- **Deer** teaches the beauty of alertness without anxiety—the fine line between presence and hypervigilance.
- **Owls** hold stillness like a sacred art. Waiting, watching, knowing when to act and when to remain unseen.
- **Ants** embody persistence. They do not question the size of the obstacle—they simply keep going.
- **Dogs** are fluent in joy, greeting each moment with full-body enthusiasm.
- **Butterflies** are reminders that transformation is messy, vulnerable, and exquisitely necessary.

Each one offers a mirror—not of who we pretend to be, but who we are underneath the noise.

This chapter is an invitation to see animals not as background characters, but as teachers. As guides. As quiet, unassuming whispers from the natural world saying, *slow down, be here.*

Lessons from the Trail

I remember pausing once on a forest trail, mid-step, because a barred owl had landed silently on a branch just above me. It was larger than I expected, majestic, unmoving, eyes round and deep like pools of knowing. We held a gaze at what felt like minutes, suspended in quiet communion. I didn't move. Neither did the owl.

We shared a moment—me rooted in wonder, it in stillness. It was as if the forest held its breath too. No rustling, no birdsong, no breeze. Just two beings existing in full presence.

And in that suspended stillness, I felt something settle inside me. Not a thought, not a realization, just a calm, a recognition. The kind that arrives wordlessly, and leaves something behind.

The owl didn't need to say anything. It didn't move to prove its power. It simply *was*. And that was enough.

Animals remind us that we do not have to *earn* our existence.

We do not need to perform to be worthy of pause.

We are allowed to rest. To feel. To breathe.

They model embodiment—being fully in their bodies, aware of the world, alert without panic, moving through space with the full knowledge that they belong here. Their stillness isn't passive, it's wise.

Joy in the Wild

Some animals teach us how to play—and remind us just how deeply we need it.

I once stood beside a quiet stream, completely captivated by a pair of otters moving through the water like it was an extension of their bodies. They twisted and dove, circled and chased, flipping onto their backs and nuzzling each other in a blur of playful motion. It was as if joy itself had taken form—light, instinctive, alive.

There was no goal.

No competition.

No finish line.

Just movement for the sake of delight.

And watching them, something shifted in me. I felt a kind of ache—not sadness, but recognition. It made me ask:

When was the last time I moved like that? Not to exercise. Not to burn calories or track steps. But simply to feel alive?

We often forget that play isn't a luxury. It's a reset. A way the nervous system rebalances itself after stress. A state where creativity returns, laughter becomes easier, and the body finds its way back to safety. Play disarms fear. It opens the door to presence.

But somewhere along the way, many of us stop playing. We replace spontaneity with structure. We trade movement for productivity. We unlearn ease.

And yet, animals never forget.

They roll in grass. Chase shadows. Flap wings just because. They leap, sprawl, pounce, and purr—not to impress or compete—but because it *feels good.* Even adult animals play. And not just when life is easy. In fact, play often shows up *alongside* risk, uncertainty, and change—as a natural counterweight to fear.

Joy, like grief, is a full-body experience. And animals know how to make room for both.

Even in our hardest seasons, joy is still available.

Sometimes it slinks, barks, climbs, or buzzes.

Sometimes it scampers up a tree. Sometimes it lands on your windowsill. It often shows up unannounced—if we're paying attention.

And joy never hurries. It invites.

In the wild, joy isn't framed or filtered. It just is.

Alive. Playful. Undeniable.

And deeply, deeply necessary.

Returning to Instinct

These animal teachers do not give us instructions; they give us reflection.

They don't ask us to copy them.

They invite us to remember ourselves.

The version of us that trusts our gut. That stops when tired. That leaps when ready. That finds nourishment in the sun and shade alike.

You do not need to speak the language of the wild to learn from it. You simply must watch.

To listen. To be.

In a world that asks us to constantly *do*, animals teach us how to simply *be*.

To rest when the day is done.

To move only when it's time. To respond, not react.

In their presence, we remember ours.

In their rhythm, we remember that we are animals, too.

Closing Reflection

Let animals be your quiet teachers.

Let the squirrel remind you to move with purpose.

Let the owl show you how to wait.

Let the deer teach you how to be both alert and soft.

Let the dog remind you that joy is sacred.

Let the otter invite you to play again.

Watch closely. Not to analyze, but to remember.

You are not separate from these rhythms. You are part of them.

You are not behind or broken, you are simply being asked to return to something ancient, something wise, something already inside you.

Let your days carry more instinct, more noticing, more trust in your own breath and body. Let your movements be rooted. Let your pauses be holy.

Because to be alive is not just to survive.

It is to *feel* your life from the inside out. Just like the animals do.

And when in doubt, look at them. They will not speak. But they will show you the way back to yourself.

Chapter 19: Nature and Grief

Grief does not ask for permission.

It does not wait for the right time or a proper setting. It arrives unannounced, folding itself into the body like fog—slow, heavy, and hard to escape. It touches everything without explanation. Some days it's sharp and overwhelming, and others, it's a dull hum in the background of your breath.

And in those moments, words often fail. The right ones don't come. The wrong ones echo too loudly. But nature, in its quiet, in its presence, seems to be understood without needing anything explained.

A forest does not flinch at sorrow.

A river does not rush you forward.

The sky does not ask you to feel better.

Instead, nature holds space—gently, without judgment. It lets you unravel in the company of something vast, rooted, and real. It does not need to know your story to offer you shelter.

There is comfort in walking among trees that have withstood seasons of loss and renewal. Their branches, once bare, are full again. They have let go without resistance, endured the long stillness of winter, and still, they reach again. In the life cycle of trees, there is no shame in shedding. The process of letting go is integral to personal growth and development.

We forget this sometimes—that grief is not a sign that we've broken, but a sign that we've loved.

When Grief Finds Nature

After my mother died, I didn't seek healing—I sought stillness. I found myself walking to the nearest park almost daily. I didn't plan it. I just started walking. I didn't want advice or conversation. I wanted a place where I could cry without explanation. Where I could sit in silence and let the weight in my chest settle without having to make it make sense.

Those trees became my silent companions. They didn't try to lift the grief, but they didn't recoil from it either. They stood still, offering me their presence, and in that presence, I felt less alone.

Grief was no less real in that park. But it was more bearable.

I could let it out into the open air.

I could lean my sorrow against the trunk of a tree and feel something steady lean back.

A trail becomes a kind of prayer.

Each step is a heartbeat, a grounding rhythm when everything else feels scattered.

A beach becomes a journal. The waves take what you cannot say and return only hush. Mountains become mirrors—weathered, unmoved by the storm, yet shaped by it all the same.

Even decay, in nature, holds dignity. Fallen branches become shelter for animals. Wilted leaves feed the soil. What is lost becomes part of something new. In the wild, nothing is wasted.

And maybe in our sadness, neither are we.

The Unexpected Visitors

You do not need answers in nature.

You do not need to explain your tears to the trees or justify your stillness to the sky.

You simply need to show up—to walk, to breathe, to cry, to be.

Nature does not fix grief.

It accompanies it.

And sometimes, that is more powerful than fixing.

Then one day, something changed.

I was sitting near a lake, deep in my own thoughts, when a loud honk shattered the quiet. A goose—bold and absurd—was strutting directly toward me, flapping its wings with righteous confidence. I tried to sidestep. It blocked me. I moved again. It marched forward, chest puffed, as if to say, *this is my territory now.*

I laughed. For the first time in days—maybe weeks—I laughed. Not a polite chuckle, but a real, surprised, belly-deep laugh.

That goose—unapologetic, ridiculous, entirely itself—cracked something open in me. Not to dismiss the grief, but to remind me that life was still here. Still strange. Still beautifully unpredictable. Even in sorrow, life was capable of delight.

Sometimes healing looks like a goose chase.

Sometimes nature holds our pain in one hand and offers absurd, feathered joy in the other.

Not to erase the grief, but to interrupt it just long enough to remind us:

We are still alive.

And being alive still includes laughter.

Grief and joy are not opposites.

They coexist.

They share a body.

They take turns at the front of the heart.

Nature knows this. It's written in every season.

Closing Reflection

Grief is not something to conquer—it is something to carry. And nature offers its hands.

It says: *Come sit beside me. No words are needed.*

It says: *You don't have to be okay to be welcome here.* It says: *Let your sadness breathe under the sky.*

When your chest feels too heavy, lean into a tree that has survived storms.

When your heart aches with absence, let the river remind you that love always moves forward—even when it's quiet.

When you feel emptied, watch how the earth still makes room for what's been lost, and somehow, keeps growing.

Nature does not ask you to be strong.

It only asks you to stay close.

To let yourself be held in something older than sorrow, deeper than words.

Let yourself grieve among the trees.

Let the wind carry the pieces.

Let joy surprise you when it is ready.

You do not need to rush.

You do not need to move on.

You only need to keep moving with.

And when you are ready, the world will still be here—soft, vast, rooted—and waiting to walk with you.

Chapter 20: The Wisdom of Tending

Pick up the watering can. Gently prune what no longer grows. Whisper if you feel moved to—plants don't ask for perfection. They respond instead to consistency, to nearness, to the quiet rhythm of care.

Tending to a plant may seem like a small act, but it is more than maintenance, it is a gesture of devotion. A humble promise: *I will keep showing up.* Even when the soil looks dry. Even when growth isn't visible. Even when you doubt yourself. Tending is not loud or immediate. It is slow faith in action.

With each return to the windowsill or garden bed, you begin to witness the quiet miracles: tiny buds at the edge of a stem, a leaf turning toward the light, roots stretching invisibly below the surface. These changes are rarely dramatic—but they are real. They are life unfolding in their own time.

And within this quiet tending lies deeper wisdom.

The Plant Teaches Us

A plant does not rush its blooming.

It does not question the pace of its own unfolding.

It simply leans into its own rhythm—resting, rooting, reaching—without apology.

And in tending to its needs, we begin to hear the gentle echo of our own. We start to soften the parts of us hardened by expectation, by urgency, by self-judgment. We begin to mirror what we are caring for: patient, steady, alive.

Because while we may think we're helping the plant grow, something in us is growing, too. Every time we return to water, to check the leaves, to turn the pot toward the sun—we're also returning to ourselves. To the practice of presence. To the sacred art of not giving up.

Tending Is a Mirror

To tend is to remember that care—simple, imperfect, faithful—changes everything.

As you water, you soften.

As you show up, you learn to let go of control.

As you observe, you begin to trust in things unseen roots forming, strength building, life preparing itself in the quiet.

Growth is not always dramatic. Sometimes it is so subtle that we only notice it in retrospect. A new leaf unfurls where we thought the branch had stopped trying. A little more breath enters your chest in a moment of peace you didn't expect. Tending invites us to pay attention to these shifts. To measure transformation in presence rather than performance.

We often imagine healing as an upward arc—quick, linear, clear. But tending teaches us a deeper truth: healing is slow, circular, and sometimes invisible. It is not measured in speed, but in staying.

And so, we keep watering. We keep showing up. We keep listening.

The Forgotten Pot

I remember a time I came across a neglected pot of soil on a back porch—abandoned after a move. At first glance, it seemed lifeless: cracked dirt, faded leaves, dried stems bent like question marks. I had no reason to expect anything. In fact, I'd never considered myself someone who could keep a plant alive.

But something in me decided to try. I watered it lightly. Set it where the morning light could find it. Checked it daily, even when I was sure it would never change.

And then one day—quietly, without warning, a tiny green shoot broke through the surface. Delicate, curved, barely visible. But undeniably alive.

It didn't arrive with flourish. It didn't announce itself. It simply emerged, because conditions had become just safe enough to try again.

In that moment, I saw myself in that fragile stem. I saw the version of me that had gone quiet. The parts that had grown dormant—not out of weakness, but because they were waiting. Waiting for gentleness. Waiting for enough care to believe it was safe to begin again.

That single sprout became more than just a plant. It became proof. That what looks barren is not necessarily broken. That growth can happen slowly, quietly, beneath the surface. That tending is not wasted even when results are invisible—because something is always responding.

Even in stillness. Even in silence.

What Tending Awakens

The parts of us that go quiet when ignored don't vanish. They retreat, protectively, into silence. But when we bring the smallest acts of care—time, attention, warmth—they begin to unfold again. They stretch. They breathe. They reach for light.

Tending is not about control. It is not about forcing something to grow. It is about creating the conditions in which growth *can* happen. Whether it's a leaf, a part of your spirit, or a relationship—you do not make it thrive. You make it *possible* to thrive.

And that shift in perspective is everything.

You begin to notice how care changes you. How your voice softens when you speak to yourself. How your nervous system settles with each small act of ritual. How your sense of worth isn't built on outcomes, but on your willingness to stay in relationship with your life.

It's easy to overlook these moments. But they matter. They are signals of quiet transformation.

You get out of bed on a harder day. You pause to take a breath before reacting. You let yourself rest instead of pushing. These are the new leaves of your own becoming.

A Sacred Reframe

Tending reorients our sense of time. It reminds us that what is slow is not stuck. That what is quiet is not unimportant. That what is not visible may still be vital.

It shifts us from performance to presence.

So often, we ask ourselves to bloom constantly. But nature never blooms all year long. It rests. It roots. It prepares. You are allowed to do the same.

Tending is a form of prayer—spoken not in words, but in action. It says: *I believe in what I cannot see yet.*

It says: *I will keep showing up.*

It says: *You are worth caring for.*

Closing Reflection

To tend is to believe in life before there's proof.

To water the soil and trust something will come.

To return with love, even when nothing appears to change.

Every act of tending—whether it's for a plant, a part of yourself, or a relationship that needs healing—is a radical gesture of faith. Of hope. Of quiet commitment.

Let the lessons of tending live in you.

Let them remind you that slow growth is still growth.

That care doesn't need to be perfect to be powerful.

That attention, offered regularly and gently, can change everything.

You do not have to bloom all at once.

You only need to turn, again and again, toward the light.

And trust that one day soon, something green will break the surface— and you will remember: you were growing all along.

Chapter 21: Making Nature Personal

Nature does not have to be remote to be meaningful. It does not need to look like a national park or require hours of hiking. Sometimes, it is the tree you pass on your way to work. The sunlight on your kitchen floor. The potted herb by your sink. Nature is not a destination—it is a relationship. And like any relationship, it becomes richer the more personally we engage with it.

This chapter is an invitation to make your connection to the natural world uniquely yours.

Maybe you find comfort in watching the sky each morning, tracking the colors and clouds like familiar moods. Maybe you feel most grounded sitting beside a neighborhood stream, listening to its small but steady voice. Perhaps you keep a nature journal, sketching leaves or noting when the first crocus blooms. You may even find yourself drawn to a particular flower, stone, or tree—not for any logical reason, but because it feels like a friend.

There is no right way to do this.

The key is noticing what draws you in—and leaning toward it.

Pay attention to what soothes you, what stirs something inside you, what makes you breathe a little easier. That is your doorway. That is where your personal relationship with nature begins.

Make rituals out of ordinary moments. Sit in the same spot through different seasons and notice how the light changes. Name the birds or trees you see often. Keep a favorite stone in your pocket. Leave your phone behind during one short walk each week. Let your walks become less about distance and more about discovery.

The more personal it becomes, the more powerful it feels.

Because this is not just about reconnecting with nature, it is about remembering yourself within it. Noticing what softens, what awakens, what feels true when you are not performing or rushing. Nature becomes not just a place to visit, but a companion. A witness. A mirror.

And the more you return to it, the more you begin to trust that you, too, are a living part of the world—wild, wise, and worthy of care.

So let it be personal. Let it be imperfect. Let it be yours.

Maybe your ritual is talking to the moon when you cannot sleep. Maybe it is whispering gratitude to a tree as you pass by. Maybe it is planting something just to watch it grow or sitting with your back against a wall warmed by the sun. Maybe it is nothing more than pausing to notice the way light plays on a puddle or how shadows move across your bedroom wall.

These gestures may seem small, but they become anchors. Invitations back to the moment. To yourself. To what matters.

And for some, nature becomes personal through the lens of a camera. Photography is its own kind of noticing. It asks you to look more closely, to pause long enough for light and shadow to speak. It is a way of saying, "I see this. I honor this." Whether you are capturing the curve of a leaf, the reflection in a puddle, or the way golden light hits the bark of a tree is not about the perfect shot. It is about the act of witnessing.

Sometimes, it is in the process of framing a subject that we discover what we really value. You might crouch lower to capture the texture of moss on stone and realize you have not slowed down like this in days. You might wait for the right moment of light on a flower's petal and notice how your breathing calms. Photography becomes a way to see what is been there all along but overlooked—a doorway into presence.

And over time, the camera roll becomes more than a collection of images. It becomes a journal. A reflection of what moved you, what called your attention, what you chose to celebrate. The way the fog rolled in that morning. The feather you found. The colors of a late summer sky. A dandelion seed caught in a spiderweb, backlit by evening sun. The delicate pattern of frost on your windshield. These are not just snapshots—they are echoes of your presence in the world.

Each image becomes a reminder of a time when you paused long enough to see. To notice. To connect. When you scroll through them later, you are not just reviewing photos; you are revisiting states of mind. Glimpses of quiet. Proof that beauty was there—and that you were, too. These are moments that tether you to the now. And to the version of yourself who was paying attention.

You do not have to be a professional. Even with a phone in your hand, you can practice seeing. Framing. Paying attention. It is less about technique and more about intention, about slowing down long enough to truly witness the world around you. That moment when you crouch to catch sunlight filtering through a leaf or wait patiently for a dragonfly to land? That is presence. That is reverence.

In this way, photography transforms from mere documentation to a form of devotion. A way of saying, "You matter" to the moss, to the sky, to the subtle changes in light. A way of honoring the moment not just with your lens, but with your attention. A love letter to the beauty that is already here, quietly unfolding all around you. It turns everyday moments into sacred ones, framing not just the scene—but the soul of experience.

Because when we personalize our connection to nature, we do not just heal—we remember that we belong. We remember that we are not outsiders in this living world, but a part of its breath, its rhythm, its unfolding story. That tree you return to, the birdsong you now recognize, the light you catch just before dusk—all of it becomes a conversation, a connection, a thread tying you back to what is real and enduring.

And in a world that so often pulls us away from our center—with noise, with urgency, with endless distraction, that remembering is everything.

Closing Reflection

Your connection to nature does not have to look like anyone else's. It does not have to be grand, structured, or shared online. It just must be real—for you. Whether it is through soil on your hands, photos on your phone, or the stillness you find sitting under a tree, what matters is that it brings you back to yourself.

Keep looking for what catches your eye. Keep returning to what calms your breath. Let your life be filled with small rituals of noticing, of honoring, of slowing down.

Because every time you step outside or look out a window or catch the scent of pine, rain, or jasmine—you are in conversation with the living world.

And in that conversation, you are not just hearing nature.

You are hearing yourself.

You are home. It is not just grounding; it is liberating. It is how we reclaim ourselves.

Chapter 22: Nature as a Mirror

Sometimes, the way the landscape looks is how we feel.

A fog that lingers low across the hills can feel like the confusion we can't name. The brittle quiet of bare branches in winter might echo our own seasons of emptiness. The first stretch of golden light after a storm feels exactly like hope returning after a long, dark ache.

Nature speaks to us—not in words, but in resonance. It doesn't explain or analyze. It doesn't fix. It reflects.

You may walk under a gray sky and feel your own weariness looking back at you. You may see the soft bloom of moss on stone and feel the hush of stillness within your chest. A gust of wind might swirl through the street and stir something you thought had settled. A sudden bloom might surprise you—just like the unexpected joy that occasionally rises despite everything else.

This is not a coincidence. It's kinship.

Nature mirrors us in ways we don't always understand, and that's what makes it sacred. A language is older than reason, more intimate than dialogue. A kind of knowing that doesn't ask for articulation.

A slow river reflects how grief moves in us—not linear, not fast, but always onward. The cracked bark of an old tree reminds us that aging is not erosion, it is endurance. The sky at dusk, awash in color, reminds us that endings can be soft, not just sharp.

These are not metaphors we impose on the world.

They are metaphors that find us—because something in us is still fluent in nature's quiet language.

Nature Doesn't Judge

There is something deeply healing about being mirrored without critique.

When we bring our emotions to the natural world, they are received without resistance.

The forest does not flinch at our sorrow.

The ocean does not turn away from our fear.

The sun rises each day—unconcerned with whether we feel whole, hurting, or anything in between.

In everyday life, we're often met with feedback, advice, or expectations—whether we ask for it or not. But nature doesn't operate that way. It doesn't try to interpret or improve our emotions. It just makes room for them.

When we bring our feelings—grief, fear, anger, exhaustion—into the natural world, they're not met with discomfort or judgment. The forest doesn't flinch at your sadness. The ocean doesn't pull away from your fear. The wind doesn't try to cheer you up.

Nature simply allows you to be exactly where you are.

You can sit quietly under a tree with something too heavy to explain, and it won't ask for reasons. It won't tell you to move on. It will just stay. Quiet. Still. Present.

This kind of presence is powerful because it's rare. In our fast-paced, solution-focused culture, there's pressure to feel better quickly or make sense of pain. But sometimes, we don't need to fix anything, we just need a place to feel what's true.

And nature offers that space.

It doesn't need words.

It doesn't rush the process. It just holds steady.

In that steadiness, something begins to shift.

Not because your sadness disappears—but because it's no longer held in isolation. You're not alone in it anymore.

Nature doesn't ask you to be okay. It just stays with you, quietly reminding you that you're still part of something larger—even when everything feels uncertain.

That's the healing.

Not the solution, but the space.

Nature holds us with an even hand. It does not demand that we shift or improve. It does not cheerlead or offer platitudes. It simply stays. Present. Quiet. Unmoving in its willingness to witness.

And in that quiet presence, something eases—not because your sorrow vanishes, but because it is witnessed, and you are no longer holding it all by yourself.

Seeing Ourselves in the Landscape

A field left wild and tangled might reflect our own sense of disorder. A sky torn with lightning may look like the moment before we break open. A flower blooming in cracked pavement might speak to the part of us that is still growing, even when it shouldn't be possible.

Nature reminds us that contradiction is not failure. It is life. Fragility and strength can coexist. Stillness and storm can both be true. The web that glimmers with dew is both delicate and enduring. The mountain that seems immovable was once molten fire.

You do not have to have it all figured out. Nature doesn't. It just changes, responds, adapts—and thrives.

And so can you.

Reflections in Motion

There are days when simply stepping outside puts you into

conversation with something wiser.

You watch birds gather and scatter, and feel your own longing mirrored in their migration. You see how branches bend in the wind and recognize that strength is not in rigidity—but in the ability to yield without breaking.

When you feel overwhelmed, watch how the clouds shift shape without resistance.

When you feel fractured, notice how water moves around obstacles without losing its flow. Even frozen ground gives way eventually to thaw.

There is nothing you can feel that nature cannot hold.

Let Nature Meet You Where You Are

Let yourself be seen—not for your performance, not for your composure, but for your presence.

You can bring your grief to the waves. You can bring your anxiety to the wind. You can bring your uncertainty to the forest floor. The earth does not turn away.

You do not need to narrate your feelings in nature. You simply need to show up. Be in the weather. Be in the moment. Let your body exist without needing to produce, explain, or perfect.

There is healing in being mirrored without being judged.

There is wisdom in being reflected on to yourself—without distortion, without pressure.

You Are Not Alone

The moon knows something about cycles. The tide knows what it means to retreat and return. The tree knows how to stand still while changing completely.

Even the silence of a stone is not empty, it is patient.

These are our teachers. Our mirrors. Our kin.

Nature does not just reflect who you are, it reflects who you are becoming. It reminds you of your belonging. That you, too, are cyclical. That you, too, are allowed to rest. That you, too, can begin again.

Closing Reflection

Let nature mirror you—not only when you're centered, but when you're tangled, hurting, lost, or uncertain. The earth does not require clarity to be present with you. It does not demand answers to offer comfort.

When you feel scattered, look at the shifting sky.

When you feel raw, rest your hand on the rough bark of an old tree. When you feel tender, trace the delicate lines of a leaf.

Whatever you are holding, there is room for it here.

Let the natural world echo the quiet truths inside you, the ones that don't need to be spoken to be understood. In doing so, you may find not only reflection, but refuge. You may find that you are not broken, only human. Not lost, only in motion.

And when you are ready, the earth will still be here mirroring your strength, your softness, and your capacity to begin again.

You don't have to explain it.

You don't have to name it.

You only have to feel it.

And let the earth feel with you.

Chapter 23: Sacred Smallness

Sometimes, the most sacred things are the smallest.

A cluster of dew on a blade of grass. The precise balance of a bee on a wildflower. The spiral etched into a snail shell. These tiny miracles do not cry out to be seen, but when we do see them—when we pause long enough to really notice—something within us shifts. We begin to understand that life doesn't whisper because it is insignificant. It whispers because it trusts you're listening.

In a world obsessed with expansion—bigger goals, bigger platforms, bigger dreams— nature gently reminds us: small is not less. Small is where magic lives. It is layered, complex, quiet, and deliberate. A single acorn holds the blueprint for an entire forest. A mushroom grows from the shadows of decay, feeding the roots of trees. A patch of moss turns stone into softness.

Nothing in the natural world questions its worth based on visibility or scale. Why should we?

The Wisdom of the Overlooked

Paying attention to smallness is an act of rebellion in a culture addicted to spectacle. It's a spiritual posture, a reorientation from striving to presence. When we slow down enough to notice the filigree of frost on a windshield, or the way light drapes over a leaf, we begin to perceive beauty that has always been there—but was waiting for us to arrive with open eyes.

This shift is not about aesthetics. It is about healing. Because when we tune into the intricacies of the world around us, we begin to recognize our own inner terrain—our texture, our rhythms, our worthiness—not in spite of our smallness, but because of it.

Small gestures—pausing before speaking, offering a quiet kindness, planting a seed— become sacred acts. These micro-moments are the mycelial threads of a meaningful life, the quiet scaffolding beneath everything visible.

Rituals Rooted in the Everyday

Sacred smallness invites ritual. Not the grand, ceremonial kind (though those have their place), but the daily devotions woven into how we move through the world.

Ritual can be as simple as stepping outside each morning barefoot, feeling the texture of the ground beneath you. It can be the way you greet the same tree on your walk, the way you breathe deeper when you see the moon rise, or the soft ritual of tending to a windowsill garden. You do not need a reason. You just need to notice.

The power of ritual lies in repetition. In return, in allowing something ordinary to become extraordinary through the quality of your attention. As you make these tiny, intentional acts part of your life, they begin to nourish something far beyond your five senses, they nourish your sense of self.

And in doing so, they also reconnect you to the living world not as something outside of you—but something you're actively a part of.

The Camera as a Sacred Tool

For many, the lens becomes a bridge. Photography, especially in natural spaces, is not merely about capturing what is seen. It is a devotional practice of observation. A Stillness. A reverent pause.

The moment you kneel to frame the curve of a petal or the way mist curls between branches, you're not just making art—you're practicing presence. You're saying, "These matters. This moment matters." And in the act of witnessing, you become more alive in the world.

Photography teaches you to seek. To wait. To trust the light. And over time, the photos you take become more than mementos. They become breadcrumbs of memory, each image marking a moment where you were fully here.

The fog along a mountain ridge. A feather on the sidewalk. A dragonfly mid-flight. These are not just things you saw, they are fragments of who you were when you were most awake to life.

You don't need fancy equipment. You don't need training. You just need the willingness to look longer, and to care.

A Personal Path to Reverence

Sacred smallness is deeply personal. No one can define what draws your attention or calms your breath. Maybe for you, it's the smell of jasmine at dusk. The color of sky before a thunderstorm. The flicker of moth wings near a porch light. These are not distractions. These are invitations. They are threads pulling you gently back to yourself.

You might find your ritual in moon-gazing, or in the rhythm of waves, or in the single tree outside your office window that changes slowly, day by day, while the rest of the world rushes past. You might find it in a tiny shell you carry in your pocket. Or in a rock garden you tend with no real purpose other than to bring you peace.

Whatever it is, lean toward it. Let it teach you how to stay.

Because the beauty of this path is that it doesn't require transformation. It simply asks for return. A return to noticing. To listen. To being right here.

Quiet as a Form of Knowing

Smallness is often equated with silence—but silence is not emptiness. It is a form of knowing. A form of being.

The more you practice sacred smallness, the more you start to hear the things that once went unnoticed. The rustle of wind in branches. The soft percussion of rain. The unspoken way the light shifts when someone you love enters the room. You learn to tune into the subtleties. And this tuning in, this sensitivity, becomes a kind of strength.

You become less reactive and more receptive. Less hurried and more whole.

In a culture that rewards volume and velocity, to be quiet is to be radical. To be soft is to be strong. And to love small things is to live in a different kind of abundance—one that does not deplete you but restores you.

The Sacred is Here

Sacred smallness reminds us that nature does not have to be remote to be holy. It does not need a summit or a stamp of wilderness approval. It might be the herb on your windowsill. The weed grows through a crack in the sidewalk. The pattern the clouds make as you wait at a stoplight.

Nature isn't a destination, it's a relationship, one that deepens with presence and care.

When that connection becomes personal, everything shifts.

You no longer stand apart from the world; you recognize yourself as part of its living tapestry.

The bird outside your window becomes a familiar voice. The dirt beneath your nails becomes belonging.

The ordinary transforms into something sacred—because you've decided to see it that way. And what we choose to truly see, we cannot help but honor.

Closing Reflection

Let your sacred be small.

Let your connection be quiet.

Let your rituals be simple and imperfect and yours.

You do not need incense or silence or sweeping views. You do not need perfect words or a perfectly still mind.

You only need presence—the kind that hums beneath the surface of ordinary things.

There is no benchmark for reverence.

No standard for worth.

The act of noticing is enough. The act of pausing is holy.

Each moment you choose to *see*—to slow down, to wonder, to care—is a thread tying you gently back to the earth, and to yourself.

The way you bend toward beauty, even on your hardest days, is a kind of prayer. A prayer not made of words, but of willingness. Of attention.

Of the courage it takes to keep your heart open in a world that rushes you past it all.

So, hold the feather.

Greet the tree.

Frame the sunlight with your lens or your breath.

Mark it.

Make it matter.

Let it be enough.

You are not lost, you're paying attention.

And that, more than anything, is the path back to yourself.

Again and again, through the quiet, through the small, through the sacred that asks nothing but you are noticing.

Conclusion: Returning Home — The Future of Nature in Urban Life

We are living through a time of constant motion—digitally connected, mentally overstimulated, and physically removed from the natural rhythms that once supported us. Cities are growing. Screens are multiplying. Daily life is faster, louder, and more crowded than ever before.

And yet, something in us is starting to be remembered.

Throughout this book, we've explored what science, practice, and personal experience all affirm: that the natural world has the power to regulate, restore, and reorient us. That even brief, consistent contact with nature improves mental health, immune function, sleep, focus, and resilience. And that the modern world, particularly in urban spaces, needs nature more urgently than ever.

But this return to nature isn't about escaping. It's about integration.

Nature doesn't need to live on the margins of our lives. It should be part of our cities, our routines, our healing, and our homes. Green space shouldn't be a luxury. It should be built into infrastructure, public health policy, education, and personal wellness strategies. We need parks that are walkable, windows that open, workdays that allow room for fresh air, and communities where a tree isn't a bonus expected.

We also need to shift how we relate to nature personally. Because the return isn't just systemic—it's internal.

The Return is Personal

Nature helps us return not just to place, but to ourselves.

You don't need a remote trail, a national park pass, or hours of free time. You don't need to be an environmentalist or a botanist. You just need presence. Willingness. A moment.

This book is not meant to be a blueprint or a checklist.

It is a trailhead. A compass.

A reminder of what you already know deep down.

Start where you are:

- Crack a window and listen to the wind.
- Walk outside without your phone.
- Step barefoot into your backyard or onto your balcony.
- Sit beside a plant and breathe with it.
- Look at the sky and let it be enough.

These are not grand gestures. They are honest ones.

Nature is not asking for perfection. It's asking for attention.

And when you give it—even in small doses—it gives something back:

A steadier heart. A clearer mind. A more grounded body. A feeling of home.

Because you are not separate from the natural world.

You are part of it.

You are made of the same elements, the same breath, the same soil, the same water and wind.

You are not a visitor here. You belong.

The Future We Shape

The healing we find in nature doesn't stop with us.

It ripples outward—into our homes, our communities, our systems, and our future.

When we begin to prioritize nature—individually and

collectively—we create cultures that are more resilient, more compassionate, and more sustainable. We remember that restoration is not always dramatic or visible. Sometimes it's small, local, and personal.

A walk becomes clarity.

A garden becomes connection.

A pause becomes a turning point.

The future of nature in urban life depends not only on design and policy—but on how often we each choose to look up, to step out, and to reconnect.

Let this book be the start of your own ripple.

Let it begin here.

Let it begin now.

Let it begin with you.

Final Affirmation

I am rooted in the rhythms of the Earth.

Even amid the noise, I can return to stillness.

Nature lives in me, around me, and beyond me.

I do not need to escape to find peace

I need only to notice, to breathe, and to begin again.

Closing Practices: Integrating Nature into Everyday Life

You don't need to do all of these. Start with one. Then return to the list when you're ready for more.

Daily

- Step outside for 5 minutes without your phone.
- Notice one natural detail, shadow, a breeze, a birdcall.
- Open a window and listen.
- Water the plant slowly and with attention.

Weekly

- Take a walk with no destination.
- Watch a sunrise or sunset without multitasking.
- Sit on a bench or patch of grass for at least 10 minutes.
- Do one task (coffee, reading, lunch) outdoors.

Monthly

- Visit a new green space, even if it's small.
- Forage or collect—leaves, textures, colors.
- Reflect on a seasonal change: What do you feel shifting in you?

Seasonally

- Revisiting a favorite spot to witness its changes.
- Adjust your rituals: different walks, foods, or outdoor habits in winter vs. summer.
- Create a small nature altar or shelf in your home with seasonal items (stones, pinecones, pressed flowers, shells).

Reader's Pledge: A Quiet Commitment to Reconnection

I commit to returning to nature—not as a task, but as a relationship.

I will create small, meaningful moments of reconnection in my daily life.

I understand that healing is not always instant or visible, but it deepens with presence, attention, and time.

I recognize that I am part of the natural world—not separate from it.

And I will let that remembering guide how I live, listen, rest, and move forward.

Signed: ____________________ *Date:* ________________

ABOUT THE AUTHOR

Dalia Latife is a certified Technical Project Manager, nature photographer, and founder of SkyTrail Consulting. After the loss of her mother in 2016, she began to see the world through a different lens. Grief reshaped her inner landscape, offering a stark reminder of life's fragility and drawing her closer to the quiet wisdom of the natural world. In the years that followed, she found comfort in trees, trails, and stillness—places where healing didn't need words and peace could arrive unannounced.

Later, after the unexpected end of a 19-year career with the same company, she found herself in another season of transition. Once again, nature offered steadiness—a way to listen inward, to reimagine purpose, and to begin again.

What began as a personal search for grounding became a lifelong practice of noticing, remembering, and returning. Through her writing, photography, and travels across landscapes both wild and wondrous, Dalia explores the quiet strength that lives in stillness, the resilience found in the natural world, and the sacred beauty of ordinary moments.

Based in South Florida, she continues to walk the path of reconnection—inviting others to find their way back to themselves, one breath, one trail, and one wild moment at a time. The Quiet Cure is her first book.

www.ingramcontent.com/pod-product-compliance
Lightning Source LLC
Chambersburg PA
CBHW062100270326
41931CB00013B/3159
* 9 7 9 8 9 9 9 7 2 1 6 2 4 *